the salon professional's guide to

FOOT CARE

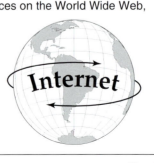

the salon professional's
guide to

FOOT CARE

BY

GODFREY MIX, DPM

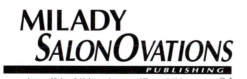

MILADY
*Salon**Ovations***
PUBLISHING

a division of Delmar Publishers, an International Thomson Publishing company I(T)P®

3 Columbia Circle, P.O. Box 12519 • Albany, New York 12212-2519

NOTICE TO THE READER

Cover Photographer: Stephane Colbert
Cover Design/Art Direction: Suzanne Nelson

Milady Staff
Publisher: Gordon Miller
Acquisitions Editor: Joseph Miranda
Project Editor: NancyJean Downey
Production Manager: Brian Yacur
Production and Art/Design Coordinator: Suzanne Nelson

COPYRIGHT © 1999
Milady Publishing
(a division of Delmar Publishers)
an International Thomson Publishing company **I T P**®

Printed in Canada

For more information, contact:
Milady/SalonOvations Publishing
3 Columbia Circle , Box 12519
Albany, New York 12212-2519

1 2 3 4 5 6 7 8 9 10 XXX 04 03 02 01 00 99

Library of Congress Cataloging-in-Publication Data

Mix, Godfrey.
    The salon professional's guide to foot care / by Godfrey Mix.
      p. cm.
    Includes bibliographical references (p. 211).
    ISBN: 1-56253-332-0
    1. Foot—Care and hygiene. 2. Toenails—Care and hygiene. 3. Beauty culture. 4. Foot—Anatomy. I. Title.
RD563.M59   1998   97-43097
617.5'85— dc21   CIP

Contents

Dedication	....	vii
Acknowledgments	....	ix
Preface	....	x
Chapter 1	**The Foot, An Overview**	1
	History	1
	Terms	6
Chapter 2	**Anatomy**	13
	Bones of the Foot	14
	Ligaments of the Foot	17
	Joint Capsule	17
	Arches of the Foot	17
	Muscles of the Lower Leg	19
	Muscles of the Foot	20
	Nerves	22
	The Blood Supply—Arteries and Veins	22
	Blood	24
	Lymphatic System	25
	Skin or Integumentary System	26
	Skin Appendages	29
Chapter 3	**Systemic Diseases and the Foot**	33
	Abusive Disease	34
	Autoimmune Disorders	36
	Arthritides	37
	Cardiovascular Disease	41
	Anemia	43
	Cerebrovascular Accident	44
	Arteriosclerosis Obliterans ("Hardening of the Arteries," ASO)	45
	Diabetes Mellitus	49

Chapter 4   Common Foot Problems 59

        The Gait Cycle 60

        Shoes 65

        Conditions of the Skin 72

        Deformities of the Foot 89

        Miscellaneous Foot Disorders 93

Chapter 5   Toenails 99

        The Normal Nail 100

        Determining Location of Disorders of the Nail Plate 106

        Toenail Disorders 109

Chapter 6   Foot Anomalies, Genetic and Medical 131

        History 131

        Genetic Anomalies 132

        Medical Anomalies 134

Chapter 7   Client History 137

        General Overview 137

        Initial Encounter Form 139

        Client Medical History 142

        Personal Evaluation 145

Chapter 8   Instruments and Equipment 151

        General Discussion 151

        Instruments 154

        Equipment 161

Chapter 9   Sanitation in the Workplace 167

        Salon Sanitation 168

        Areas of the Salon 179

Chapter 10   The Pedicure 185

        Overview 185

        Pedicure Products 188

        Pedicure Procedure 190

        Reflexology 198

Answers to Chapter Review Questions 205

Further Reading Selections 211

Appendix of Sources 215

Glossary / Index 221

DEDICATION

I dedicate this book to my wife, Laura, who has been for 37 plus years my inspiration, my love, and my greatest promoter. Also a special dedication to my mother and father, who advised me, at a very early age, that I could succeed at anything I desired if I set my mind to it. This book is direct proof of that advice. They are no longer with me in person but continue to guide me in spirit!

ACKNOWLEDGMENTS

I owe many people a debt of gratitude for helping me bring this book to final print. My wife Laura has been by my side, offering encouragement, ideas, and support when I most needed it. I am sure she is tired of reading the words I put down on paper, but she continues to do so with all the love and devotion she has given freely to me over our many years together. My daughters Jackie and Lori have always been there when I most needed them. To my mother, I thank her from the bottom of my soul. She was a teacher by profession and a teacher to her last breath. She has instilled her passion for learning and teaching within me and this book is the result. To George and Joan Beitzel and many other personal friends, too numerous to mention, you have all believed in me and continue to offer words of wisdom and assistance.

A special thanks goes to Norm Freed who 4 years ago sat down in a coffee shop with Laura and me and planted the seed that has grown into this volume. He has been my director, mentor, father confessor, and most of all a friend throughout the writing of this manuscript. He continues to inspire me to greater accomplishments.

To my many patients who have offered words of encouragement I thank you. To those of you who allowed the world to view the images of your feet in the following pages I thank you from the bottom of my heart. Without you the educational process would not be fulfilled.

The beauty professionals, particularly those nail professionals with whom I have had the privilege of coming in contact, have all contributed more to this book than they will ever know. Because of you there was a need and because of you it has been written. Your questions and desire for knowledge have encouraged me throughout. You have given my life a better focus and for this I thank you one and all.

Lastly, but by far not the least, I owe thanks to my teachers, both undergraduate and professional, for instilling in me the concepts of learning and teaching. You are too numerous to mention but I thank you all. My professors and colleagues in the profession of podiatry have helped to make the study of the human foot and the disorders affecting it my life's work. I humbly thank you for the knowledge that has enabled me to pass on to others that which you have taught me. Knowledge is a gift and to pass it on is the responsibility of those to whom it has been given.

The publisher would like to thank the following professionals for their expertise in reviewing this manuscript: Grace Francis, Vista, CA; Phyllis Mitchum, Charleston, SC; Doug Schoon, Vista, CA; and Sue Ellen Schultes, Washington, NJ.

PREFACE

This book is meant to acquaint the lay person and beauty professional with the human foot. I have attempted to use terms that are understandable to the nonmedically trained individual, and any boldfaced terms can be found in the glossary. Although this book has been written for the nail professional, chapters 1 through 6 will be of interest to those desiring to expand their knowledge concerning the foot. Chapter 1 gives a general outline of the historical development of the foot from the time fish moved from the sea to begin life on land as we know it today. As you will learn, the foot has evolved through many stages to become the unique human organ of locomotion that allows us to move about in the upright position. Subsequent chapters discuss anatomy, systemic diseases as they affect the foot, common foot problems, toenails (normal and abnormal), and some of the more common medical and genetic foot anomalies. The nail professional is advised and cautioned about providing foot services to particular clients. The remaining chapters are of particular interest to students entering the beauty industry who are studying professional foot and nail care as it relates to their field. Learning objectives will help reinforce the key points and they are called out within the text for easy reference. For beauty professionals, and more particularly the nail professional who provides foot services, this book is an excellent reference on the subject and should be in the library of every salon and school.

The human organ of locomotion is something with which I have been intimately involved for the past 30 years. My professional focus has been aimed at the disease processes of the foot and has deviated little during that time—that is until a few years ago when the practice of medicine in general and more particularly as it relates to the care of the foot became more regulated under a concept called "managed medical care." Doctors' independent decision-making capabilities became replaced by a committee-type approach to treatment. This concept, in my opinion, acts as a wedge between the doctor and the patient. Instead of being satisfying and fun, my job had become regimented and business-oriented. Needless to say for one who for many years had been having "fun" practicing independent quality medicine, as it relates to the foot, the change became extremely frustrating.

During this period my wife of 30+ years was having a hard time living with my frustrations and mood changes. At her insistence we attended a personal effectiveness training course sponsored by Lifespring, Inc. This organization allows one to bring about a shift in the ability to "think and act effectively in the face of a wider range of challenges." Because of this I was able to move outside of the imaginary box, where I felt safe, which I had created for myself practicing podiatry. It has allowed me to look beyond the specific patient-doctor relationship that I had felt comfortable with for so many years. I am now able to take a risk without the fear of failure. My involvement with the beauty industry, more particularly the manicure-pedicure branch of this industry, is my risk. This book is a part of that risk and the more I commit to paper the more certain I become that this is a successful and fulfilling undertaking.

In the back of my mind I have always believed there should be a better relationship between the pedicurist and the podiatrist when it comes to the routine care of the human foot. As I became more involved in this industry I found few resources available to the nail professional concerning the human foot. I trust that this work will help fill that void. I believe that it can be used as a basic learning tool for those who wish to understand and learn about the foot. It may also be used as a general reference for those who desire to gain understanding of a particular area of interest concerning the foot.

As I have learned from my Lifespring experience, "There are no accidents." I was meant to put my knowledge to print and if you are reading this it also is not an accident! This book is meant for you and I am sure it will serve you well. Enjoy your learning experience but most of all have fun as you do it!

— G. F. Oscar Mix, DPM

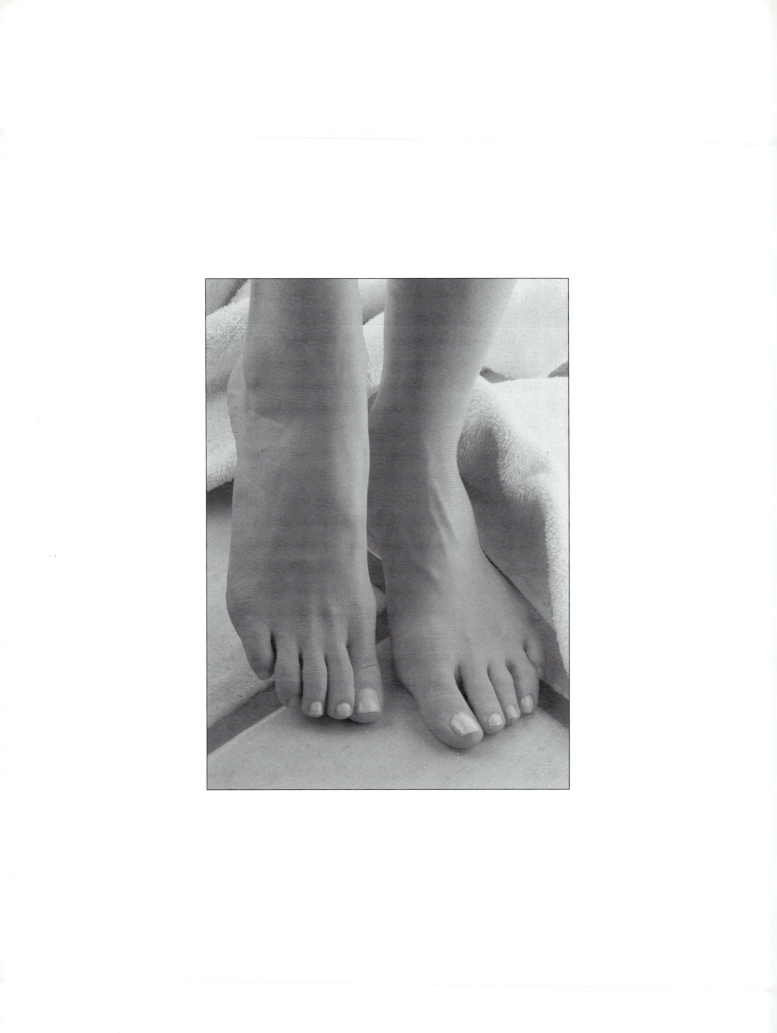

The Foot, an Overview | 1

HISTORY

The human foot is unlike any other foot on earth, and is, therefore, the most distinctly human part of our anatomy. This fact has been verified by physical anthropologists, comparative anatomists, and many other researchers. No other foot within the animal kingdom is specifically adapted for leverage to allow walking upright. Because of this adaptation, humans are the only animals to ambulate in the vertical position! This upright mode of walking places the human foot under tremendous stress. These stresses magnify the many mechanical and physical problems that providers of foot services observe. By being aware of this fact as you read through this book the causes of calluses, ingrown nails, and other commonly observed foot abnormalities will become clear.

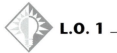
Millions of years ago as the seas began drying up, many species of fish began adapting to life on land. The paired fins of these fish had to adapt as legs to allow for movement in this new environment. Adaptations of the skeletal structures of the fins of these early fish can be traced, through fossil remains and living specimens of today, to what we now call the human foot. When the bones and soft tissues of man and other primates are compared separately and collectively, the similarities between man and the gorillas and chimpanzees are most impressive. The evaluation of fossil remains of prehistoric man demonstrates structural differences of the leg and foot, which may be looked at as intermediate changes between man and apes. *The development of the longitudinal arch in the modern day human foot has made it that specialized organ for leverage, which allows us to walk in the upright manner.* Apes do not have an arch. This makes their feet more flexible and unable to support or propel them efficiently in the upright manner.

It is estimated that the erect mode of walking first began over 3 million years ago. The footprints of early man (*hominid*) are found in fossilized mud of that era (Figure 1-1). The early prehistoric fossilized remains of *Australopithecus habilis* who existed 1.75 million years ago show the beginnings of longitudinal and transverse arches in their feet. They also exhibit a modern day great toe structure. *Homo erectus* who lived 1.5 million years ago demonstrates a more advanced arch structure. *Homo sapiens* came into the picture three to four hundred thousand years ago and fossils of that era display a foot structure as we know it today. One wonders if these early *Homo sapiens* had as many foot problems as we do today. When their feet hurt, did they hurt all over? Were they able to predict the coming of a storm when their bunion or callus began hurting? We can only guess!

What we can be sure of is the fact that much more stress was placed on the foot as we began walking upright. Small disorders of the foot became magnified because of the extra stress and weight being applied to it. Before the advent of the human foot there was no such thing as a "fallen arch!" Hammertoes and bunions were unheard of. Ingrown toenails as we know them were nonexistent. Have you ever seen an ape complain of a painful callus?

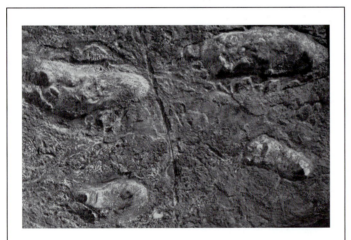

Figure 1-1 *Fossilized footprints made by two* **hominids**, *3.6 million years ago, discovered on the Laetoli plain of Tanzania. They demonstrate upright gait, and a foot with a longitudinal arch and modern day great toe positioning, almost identical to ours. (Photograph reproduced by permission of Professor Michael H. Day, Emeritus Professor of Human Anatomy, University of London.)*

Walking in the upright manner, is it worth the pain and distress that comes with it?

Foot Covering and Care

In Chapter 5 you will learn that it is thought that our ancestors of 12,000 years ago began wearing foot coverings to protect their feet from the cold. From these early foot coverings more protective shoes came into being and along with them all of the associated foot disorders. Corns, different types of fungal and yeast infections, and other types of skin irritations from the shoe materials all became apparent with the advent of shoes. Shoes also increased the need for foot care and from these humble beginnings arose the professional art of caregiving for the feet.

Egyptian tombs give us our earliest written and pictorial history of foot care. Max Müller, an Egyptologist, unearthed in a tomb, estimated to date about 2450 BC, what is probably the first known pictorial representation of a foot operation. At that time barbers also practiced as surgeons. The picture shows the patient resting his foot in front of the surgeon who is administering some type of treatment to his great toe. Reflexologists claim this picture illustrates a reflexology treatment. Whatever it illustrates, it is indeed the earliest picture of a foot being cared for.

Hippocrates (460–377 BC), the father of medicine, was the first to describe a club foot deformity. He recommended early manipulative treatment for this disorder in children and was the first to advance the use of corrective shoes for a therapeutic treatment to accommodate this deformity in adults. As time went by we find more mention of foot abnormalities in literature. Galen (130–210 AD), a Greek physician, was a prolific writer of medical literature, in which he discusses the treatment of corns, callosities, and bruised nails. Many of these problems were probably influenced by the style of footwear. In those days there were no right and left shoes. Shoes were made to please the eye of the buyer and not to fit the foot—a complaint we still hear today!

The priest-physicians of Aesculapius maintained health baths in their ancient Grecian temples. Roman baths on the other hand were not supervised by priest-physicians but seem to be modeled after them as far as services were concerned. The aqueducts of Rome provided a constant supply of fresh water to the baths, making them far superior to their counterparts in Greece. Hydrotherapy or "water cure" and massage treatments for arthritic problems were offered. The treatment of corns, calluses, and nails was also part of the services available in these surroundings. This may have been the early origins of the professional pedicurist.

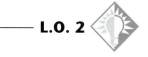

L.O. 2

Historically, the demand for foot care, whether surgical or conservative, has been in existence since the beginnings of mankind. With this fact in mind why is the common corn or callus and the ingrown toenail still such a mystery today? The answer may lie in the early recommendations for treatment of these maladies. The "Ebbers Papyrus," written 1500 years ago, promoted the application of cow fat and olive oil for the treatment of corns. Hikesios of Smyrna, born about 60 BC, recommended the application of plaster preparations to treat these lesions. Celsus, who lived during the reign of Tiberius Caesar, advocated the use of ash of willow bark, which is related to salicylic acid, a corn preparation commonly used today.

Pliney the Elder (circa 23–79 AD) proposed the use of boar or swine dung as a remedy for corns. He also suggested that "Whoever, when he sees a shooting star, soon afterwards pours a little vinegar upon the hinge of a door is sure to get rid of his corns." Paul of Aegina (615–690 AD) describes a surgical approach to the corn by directing "Wherefore having scarified around the clavus or corn and taking hold of it with a forceps we cut it out by the roots with a sharp-pointed scalpel or lancet for bleeding. So in order that it may not grow again, apply heated cauteries." The use of brass filings, old soap, and oil were recommended by the Anglo-Saxons as a treatment for "hangnail."

The list goes on and on! Corns were thought to be a "disturbance of the humors of the skin." The actual mechanical traumatic cause was missed completely! These myths go on today. The over-the-counter corn remedies of today were advocated centuries ago. They did not work then and they do not work today. We hear about different remedies for corns every day. (Chapter 5 discusses the corn and callus in detail.)

Foot Binding

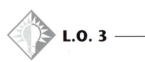 **L.O. 3**

In the not so distant past some societies made the foot a major part of their culture. For almost 1000 years, from the 11th to the 20th centuries, the Chinese practiced foot binding. This custom spread to Korea, Japan, Indochina, and even into eastern Russia. The bound foot of the female was viewed by Chinese society as being the most desirable, erotic part of the female anatomy. The "Lotus Foot," as it was called after binding, had the appearance of a lotus flower and was said to reflect the essence of the owner's personality. The smaller the foot the more desirable it became. It is thought the custom started in the palaces by the palace dancers. This suggests that the binding was originally not tight but was used to make the feet look smaller and caused the dancer to move in a mincing swaying step to maintain balance. The practice soon spread beyond the palaces and millions of Chinese women with bound feet became the perfect sexual symbols of their day. The upper classes demonstrated their wealth by being able to care for wives who could not care for themselves. The Lotus Foot was virtually impossible to walk on for any distance. Therefore, servants were hired to carry the lady wherever she went.

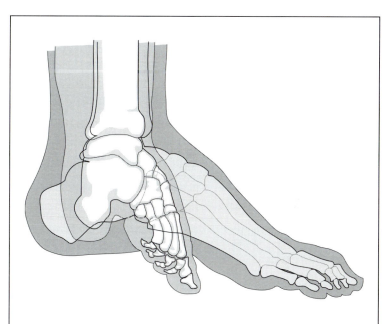

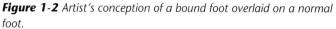

Figure 1-2 *Artist's conception of a bound foot overlaid on a normal foot.*

The process of foot binding began when the female child was about 5 years old; however, sometimes the child was 12 to 14 years old. Whatever the age, it was a painful process. It was endured because the custom was so prevalent that it became a prerequisite for a proper marriage. Large feet became a mark of a lower class or peasant background. Special and elegant footwear and shoes were developed to draw attention to the tiny feet. These shoes were custom made and were usually made small so the foot had to be compressed further to fit into them. The shoes were not necessarily comfortable but made the foot appear all that much smaller.

The practice of foot binding was finally banned in the early 20th century as part of the larger movement to emancipate and elevate the status of women. In 1895, ten women of different nationalities formed the "Natural Foot Society." Through the efforts of this society, an Anti-footbinding Edict was issued, in 1902, after which the practice gradually died out. However, the stigma of large feet still lives on today. How many women in our society think their feet are too large? Women's shoes are still made to make feet appear smaller than they actually are! Everyone complains but no one wants to wear a shoe that makes her feet look big!

Foot Fetishism

To some, the foot and the coverings of the foot are erotic objects that stimulate sexual desires. The term for this is fetish and occurs when some material object or nonsexual part of the body arouses sexual desire and may even become necessary for sexual gratification. Of all sexual fetishes the foot or shoe fetish is the most prevalent. The reasons for this are not clear. The majority of the individuals who have a foot or shoe fetish are men. The foot or shoe fetishists come from all walks of life and every segment of society. They are married or single and for the most part their fetishism is not harmful and is accepted by those close to them.

An understanding of descriptive terms is vital to providing effective care.

You should understand some of the terms used in discussing the foot or any other part of the body. This understanding becomes more important if you desire to talk to a podiatrist or other medical practitioner about a foot problem. Just as nail professionals have a language of their own so do medical professionals. To communicate with each other we must understand each other's particular language. We need to express ourselves clearly by using the proper terms correctly. The following discussion and drawings will acquaint you with some of the basic terms used to describe body parts and more particularly the parts and motions of the foot.

Anatomic Position

L.O. 4 ——— All descriptions of body parts and movements of the body are described in relation to the **anatomic position**. The anatomic position is the position that is assumed when a person stands erect with the head, eyes, and toes directed forward. The arms are by the sides of the body with the palms of the hands facing forward and the legs together (Figure 1-3). You must be able to visualize this position whenever you are talking about the relationships and motions of the foot or any body part.

L.O. 5 ——— Once the anatomic position of the body is assumed then one can describe four imaginary planes that pass through the body.

1. **Median plane**—This plane divides the body into equal left and right halves. It passes through the center of the body from front to back and from top to bottom. The median plane of the foot would pass through the middle of the third toe to the middle of the heel thus equally dividing the foot into two equal halves (Figure 1-4).

2. **Sagittal planes**—These are multiple planes that run parallel to the median plane. They differ from the median plane in that they do not divide the body or body part into equal halves (Figure 1-5).

3. **Coronal or frontal planes**—These are vertical planes that pass through the body or body part at right angles to the median plane. These planes divide the body or body part into front (*anterior*) and back (*posterior*) portions (Figure 1-6).

4. **Horizontal or transverse planes**—These planes are at right angles to both the median and coronal planes. These planes divide the part into a top and a bottom. In the foot the top is called the dorsal aspect and the bottom is the plantar aspect (Figure 1-7).

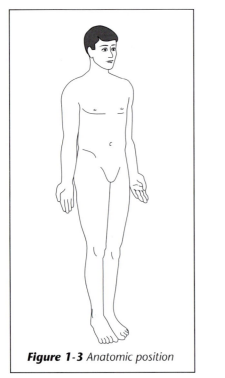

Figure 1-3 *Anatomic position*

Terms of Relationship

Other terms describe the relationship of one body part to another. Remember all of these terms assume the body to be in the anatomic position. The following terms describe the foot parts.

 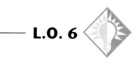

- **Dorsal**—Refers to the top of the foot, or to a part nearer to the top of the foot, i.e., the skin on the *dorsal* (top) aspect of the foot is thinner than that on the sole.

- **Plantar**—Refers to the bottom of the foot, or a part nearer to the bottom of the foot, i.e., the callus is on the *plantar* (bottom) aspect or sole of the foot.

- **Proximal**—A position or part toward the heel, i.e., the metatarsal is *proximal* to the toe.

- **Distal**—A position or part toward the toes, i.e., the toe is *distal* to the metatarsal.

- **Intermediate**—Means between two structures, i.e., the *intermediate* phalanx is a bone that lies between the proximal and distal phalanges in the toe.

- **Medial**—Toward the median plane or center of the part, i.e., the fourth toe is *medial* to the fifth toe.

- **Lateral**—Away from the median plane or center of the part, i.e., the fifth toe is *lateral* to the fourth toe.

To complicate this a bit more, some positions or parts of a foot can be related to the bones in the leg. This is particularly apparent in naming the toenail margins.

- **Tibial**—Refers to the nail margin or part of the foot toward the tibia, which is a bone of the leg. It is on the same side of the leg as the big toe. The terms tibial and medial can be used interchangeably; podiatrists generally use the term tibial in relation to a toenail margin, i.e., the *tibial* toenail margin could also be called the *medial* toenail margin.

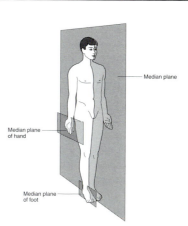

Figure 1-4 *Median plane*

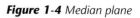
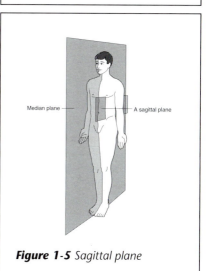

Figure 1-5 *Sagittal plane*

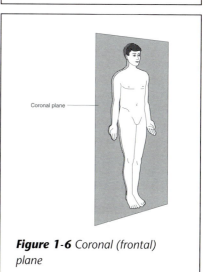

Figure 1-6 *Coronal (frontal) plane*

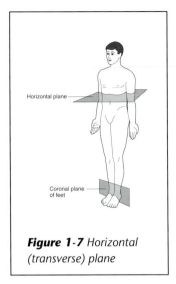

Horizontal plane

Coronal plane of feet

Figure 1-7 *Horizontal (transverse) plane*

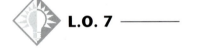

L.O. 7 ———

◆ **Fibular**—Refers to the nail margin or part of the foot toward the fibula, which is a bone on the outside or lateral aspect of the leg. It is on the same side of the leg as the little toe. The terms fibular and lateral can be used interchangeably; again podiatrists generally use the term fibular in relation to a toenail margin, i.e., the *fibular* toenail margin could also be called the *lateral* toenail margin.

Terms of Motion

The foot can move in many different directions. The following terms define the different movements of the foot.

◆ **Dorsiflexion**—A motion in the sagittal plane causing the foot or toes to move up toward the leg (Figure 1-8).

◆ **Plantarflexion**—A motion in the sagittal plane causing the foot or toes to move down or away from the leg (Figure 1-9).

◆ **Adduction**—Rotational motion of the leg in the horizontal or transverse plane causing the toes or distal aspect of the foot to move toward the median plane (Figure 1-10).

◆ **Abduction**—Rotational motion of the leg in the horizontal or transverse plane causing the toes or distal aspect of the foot to move away from the median plane (Figure 1-11).

◆ **Inversion**—The sole or plantar aspect of the foot moves in the frontal plane toward the midline or median plane of the body (Figure 1-12).

◆ **Eversion**—The sole or plantar aspect of the foot moves in the frontal plane away from the midline or median plane of the body (Figure 1-13).

◆ **Supination**—Complex triplane (taking place in three different body planes) motion consisting of simultaneous movement of the foot in the directions of adduction, inversion, and plantarflexion (Figure 1-14).

◆ **Pronation**—Complex triplane (taking place in three different body planes) motion consisting of simultaneous movement of the foot in the directions of abduction, eversion, and dorsiflexion (Figure 1-15).

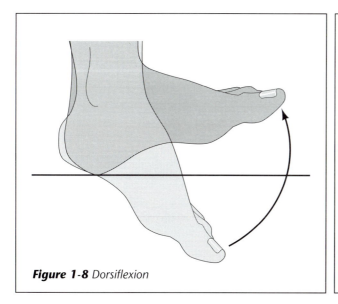

Figure 1-8 *Dorsiflexion*

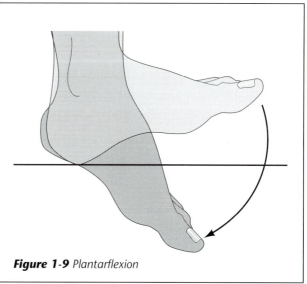

Figure 1-9 *Plantarflexion*

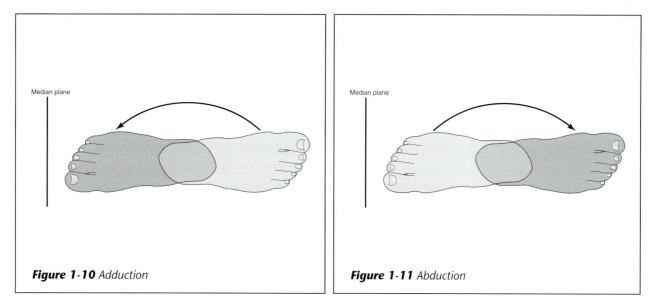

Figure 1-10 *Adduction*

Figure 1-11 *Abduction*

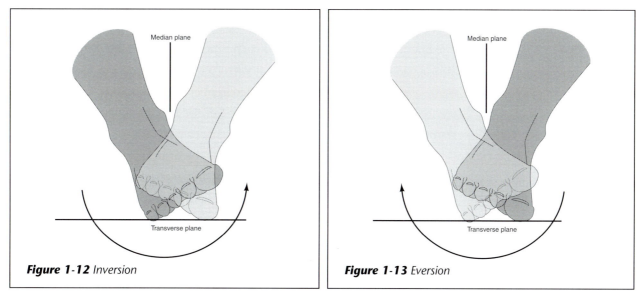

Figure 1-12 *Inversion*

Figure 1-13 *Eversion*

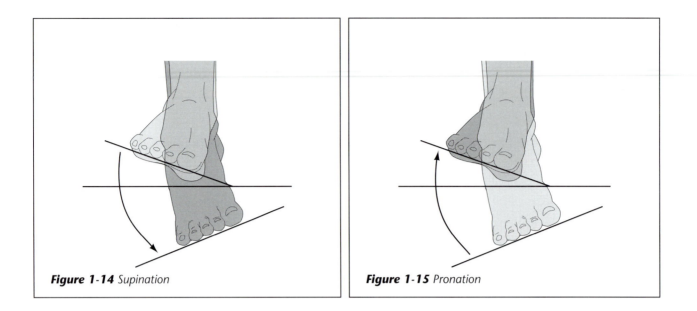

Figure 1-14 *Supination*

Figure 1-15 *Pronation*

FOOT NOTES

Our arched foot, which allows us to be the only animal to walk in the upright manner, excites many people in many different ways. The podiatrist, pedicurist, pedorthist, shoe salesperson, reflexologist, runner, anthropologist, and even the foot fetishist all look at the foot from a different point of view. We trust that the following text and chapters of this book will help you become better aquainted with this truly one of a kind organ of locomotion. Whether you use this book as a text or a reference, we are sure you will gain a better understanding regarding the subject of the human foot.

Every occupation or profession has its own particular language or set of terms that sets it apart from the others. To communicate with one another, we must understand each other's languages and terms. This becomes even more important when one specialist desires to communicate and be understood by someone in another specialty. To follow discussions in this book an understanding of the terms defined in this chapter will be a benefit to the reader.

All of these terms are defined under the assumption of the "anatomic position." By having a picture of the anatomic position in your mind, it is easy to remember how the various terms relate to the positions and locations of body parts.

QUESTIONS

1. During the process of evolution what development occurred in the human foot that allowed us to walk in the upright manner?

2. What was the bound foot of the Chinese female called?

3. The anatomic position is described as?

4. Why is it important to visualize the anatomic position?

5. The term dorsal refers to what part of the foot?

6. The term plantar refers to what part of the foot? What other term is also used for this part of the foot?

7. The tibial toenail margin is on the same side of the leg as what bone of the leg? In anatomic terms on what side of the leg is this bone located?

8. The fibular toenail margin is on the same side of the leg as what bone of the leg? In anatomic terms on what side of the leg is this bone located?

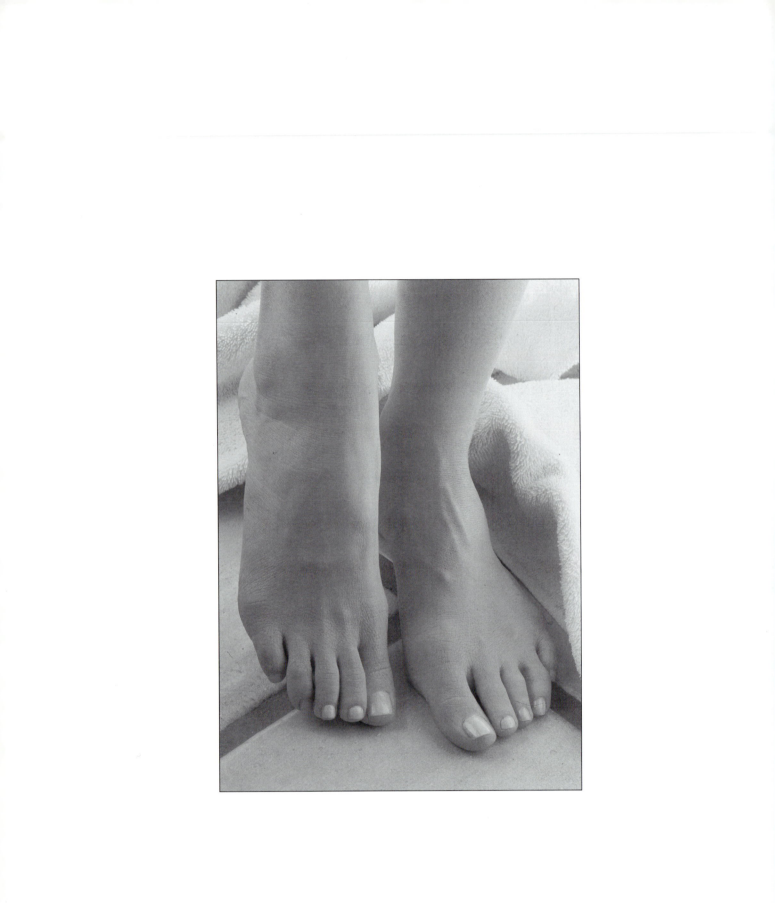

Anatomy 2

LEARNING OBJECTIVES

After studying this chapter, the reader should be able to:

1. Describe the two functions of the foot during walking.

2. Describe the three groups of bones in the foot.

3. Describe the function of the ligaments in the foot.

4. Identify the arches within the foot.

5. Describe and outline the functions of the three groups of muscles of the lower leg.

6. Describe and outline the functions of the two groups of muscles in the foot.

7. Identify the functions of the layers of plantar muscle.

8. Briefly describe the nerve supply to the foot.

9. Briefly describe the blood supply to the foot.

10. Compare and contrast arteries, veins, capillaries, arterioles, and venules.

11. Identify and describe the four parts of the blood.

12. Describe the function of lymph and the lymphatic system.

13. List five functions of the skin.

14. Describe the five layers of the epidermis.

15. Identify the two elements found in the dermis.

16. Describe the hypodermis.

17. Name the four skin appendages.

18. Describe the parts of a nail.

19. Describe the differences between sweat glands and sebaceous glands.

This chapter is not designed to make you an anatomist. It is to be used as a basis to better understand the foot and its functions. It may also be used as a reference when reading other chapters or when giving a service to your client. Other books go into much greater anatomic detail than will be discussed here and may be used if you need more detailed information on this subject.

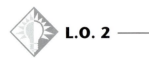

L.O. 1 ———

The human foot is a complex **organ** designed to assist us in moving from one place to another. To do this it goes through two distinct functions during the **gait cycle** (walking). At heel strike to the point where the entire foot is in contact with the surface being walked on, the foot is adapting to the surface. The adaptive phase of gait is the first function. Once the foot has adapted to the terrain it is being required to step on, it then enters its second function. The heel lifts off the weight-bearing surface and the foot propels the body forward. This is the propulsive phase of gait or the second distinct function of the foot during one step of the gait cycle.

Our feet are wonderfully adaptive and flexible, yet still function as a rigid level to move us forward

During the adaptive phase the foot must be extremely flexible to allow us to accommodate for different types of surfaces without hurting. For example, if one is walking on the sidewalk and steps on a crack or small stone, the foot should be able to adapt for that depression or elevation. Flexibility allows the foot to do this without injury, whereas if it were rigid pain or injury might result. Flexibility becomes even more important when hiking in the mountains on rough uneven surfaces where the foot must adapt to different extremes during each cycle of gait.

Once the foot has adapted to the weight-bearing surface it then must become a rigid lever to enable it to propel the body forward. If the foot remained flexible it would have a difficult time pushing us forward when we walk! In fact, many, if not the majority, of the common foot problems start during the gait cycle. If the foot fails to change from a loose bag of bones that it basically is during the adaptive phase, to a rigid structure or lever during the propulsive phase, problems such as bunions arise.

We will discuss this type of problem (biomechanical) in more detail in Chapter 4 but for now it is mentioned to demonstrate the complexity of this organ, the human foot. To understand the foot it is necessary to have a basic picture of the anatomic parts that allow it to function.

B O N E S   O F   T H E   F O O T

L.O. 2 ———

The bones of the body can be compared to the foundation of a building on which all other structures are built. Without bones to support us we would be just a pile of tissue without form or shape. The foot has 26 bones, 33 joints, and 107 ligaments holding it together. One-third of the bones of the body are contained within the feet! The 26 bones of the foot are divided into three groups—the tarsal bones, the metatarsal bones, and the phalangeal bones.

Tarsal Bones

The seven tarsal bones (Figure 2-1) extend from the heel of the foot to approximately the middle of the foot. They include some of the largest bones found in the foot. The tarsal bones are often referred to as the tarsus portion of the foot.

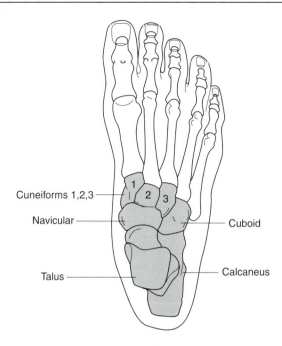

Figure 2-1 *The seven tarsal bones*

Talus. Also known as the *astragalus* or *ankle bone,* this is the second largest of the tarsal bones and basically connects the rest of the foot to the leg. It articulates (joins) with the leg bones (tibia and fibula) at the ankle, the heel bone (calcaneous), and the navicular bone.

Calcaneous. Also known as the *os calcis* or *heel bone,* this is the largest of the tarsal bones and the largest bone in the foot. It articulates with the talus and the cuboid. The joint formed between the calcaneous and talus, the subtalar joint, is the most important joint of the foot. Its proper function allows the other joints of the foot to lock (become a rigid lever) and unlock (become a loose bag of bones) between the propulsive and adaptive phases of gait.

Without the subtalar joint, our foot could not lock to be a rigid lever nor unlock to be a bag of bones.

Navicular. Also known as *the scaphoid bone,* this bone is in about the middle of the foot and on its medial (inside, or big toe) side. It articulates with the talus and the first, second, and third cuneiform bones.

Cuboid. Also known as the *os cuboideum,* this bone lies on the lateral (outside) of the foot and articulates with the calcaneous and the fourth and fifth metatarsals.

Medial Cuneiform. Also known as the *internal cuneiform,* this is the most medial of the three cuneiform bones. It articulates with the navicular, intermediate cuneiform, first metatarsal, and second metatarsal bones.

Intermediate Cuneiform. Also known as the *middle cuneiform,* this bone lies between the medial and lateral cuneiform bones. It articulates with the navicular, the medial and lateral cuneiforms, and the second metatarsal bone.

Lateral Cuneiform. Also known as the *external cuneiform,* this bone lies between the intermediate cuneiform and the cuboid. It articulates with the navicular, the intermediate cuneiform, the cuboid, and the second and third metatarsals.

Metatarsal Bones

There are five metatarsal bones (Figure 2-2). They are numbered from the medial to the lateral on the foot. They all articulate with the tarsal bones on their proximal (nearest to the heel) ends. Their distal (away from the heel) ends articulate with the toe bones. They all have similar appearances differing mainly in their lengths. The distal aspect of a metatarsal is called the *head*, the middle is the *shaft*, and the proximal part is the *base*.

First Metatarsal. This is the shortest of the metatarsal bones. It also has the greatest diameter of any of the metatarsals. When seen on an x-ray two small pea-sized bones are noticed under the head of this metatarsal. These are called sesamoid bones and can be looked at as similar to our kneecap. The sesamoids are not classified as part of the 26 true bones of the foot because of their embryologic origin. They are present for the attachment of small muscles and aid in the stabilization of the first metatarsal phalangeal (big toe) joint.

Second Metatarsal. This is the longest of the metatarsal bones.

Third Metatarsal. This metatarsal bone looks like the second metatarsal but is shorter.

Fourth Metatarsal. This metatarsal is shorter than the third metatarsal but otherwise has the same overall appearance as the second and third metatarsals.

Fifth Metatarsal. This metatarsal is shorter than the fourth metatarsal. Its head and shaft have the same appearance as the second, third, and fourth metatarsals. Its base is different in that it has an eminence (tuberosity, bump) of bone on its lateral aspect. This is called the styloid process and a muscle from the leg inserts into it. It may be seen as a "bump" on the outside of the foot on many people. It can be fractured (broken) off the metatarsal when the foot is forcibly twisted in, such as during a fall or sprain.

Phalangeal Bones

The 14 phalangeal bones (Figure 2-3) form the toes. The toes are counted from medial to lateral. The great (big) toe or hallux is the first and the little toe is the fifth. Digits two through five have three phalanges each, the proximal phalanx, the intermediate phalanx, and the distal phalanx. The

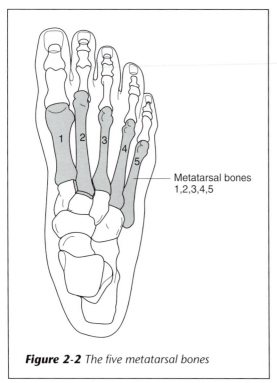

Metatarsal bones 1,2,3,4,5

Figure 2-2 The five metatarsal bones

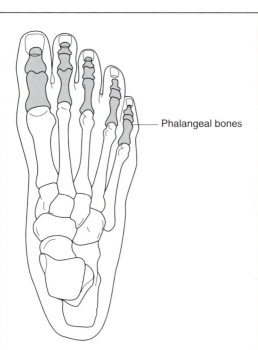

Phalangeal bones

Figure 2-3 The phalangeal bones

hallux has only two, the proximal and distal phalanx that are similar in shape but much larger than any other of the phalanges.

LIGAMENTS OF THE FOOT

The ligaments hold the bones together at their joints. They are composed of long fibrous strands and have only slight elastic qualities. You can compare a ligament, in a very loose way, to an elastic "bungee" rope. A bungee rope is composed of many small elastic rubber strands coiled together. If the bungee rope is stretched too far a few of the rubber strands will break and curl up on themselves never to reattach. A ligament if stretched too far will do much the same. A few of the strands may break and curl back on themselves. They will not stretch back out and heal end to end but will only scar across the injured area. This scar is never as strong as the original fibers of the ligament. This is what happens in a sprain, which is a partial or full tear of the ligament, and is the reason why it is sometimes said that a sprain is worse than a fractured bone. The bone will heal as strong if not stronger than it originally was, but the ligament never will. When we talk about a sprain of the ankle or foot we are really talking about a tear of the ligament in that area.

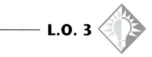 L.O. 3

Did you know your ligaments are like bungee ropes?

JOINT CAPSULE

Around and enclosing each joint is a joint capsule (Figure 2-4). The capsule is like a loose bag of tissue enclosing the joint. It is lined with a tissue called the **synovial membrane** that secretes a fluid to keep the joint lubricated. In rheumatoid arthritis the synovial membrane becomes inflamed and swollen and stops secreting the lubricating fluid. The extreme joint changes seen in rheumatoid arthritis are in part due to the changes in the lubricating mechanism of the joints.

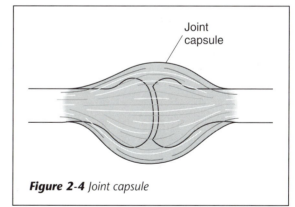

Joint capsule

Figure 2-4 Joint capsule

ARCHES OF THE FOOT

Structurally or anatomically there are four identifiable arches within the foot. The most identifiable is the *medial (inside)* **longitudinal** *arch* (Figure 2-5). It extends from the base of the great toe joint back to the heel. When one refers to a "fallen arch" this is the arch meant.

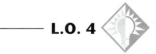 L.O. 4

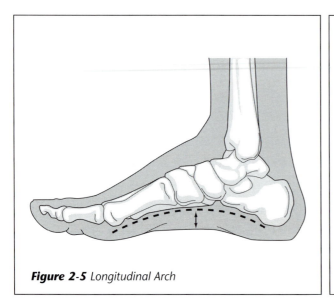

Figure 2-5 *Longitudinal Arch*

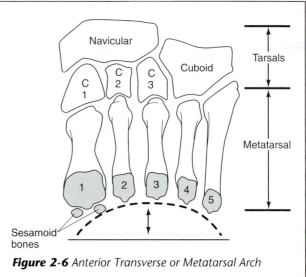

Figure 2-6 *Anterior Transverse or Metatarsal Arch*

The *metatarsal or* **anterior** *(front of the foot)* **transverse** *(medial to lateral or side to side)* arch is formed by the first through fifth metatarsal heads (Figure 2-6).

The other two arches in the foot are the *lateral (outside) longitudinal (front to back) arch* (Figure 2-7) and the **posterior** *(closer to the heel) transverse arch* (Figure 2-8). The lateral longitudinal arch extends from the base of the little toe back to the heel. The posterior transverse arch is formed by the first, second, and third cuneiform bones as well as the cuboid.

A true case of "fallen arches" is an extremely rare occurrence! The true culprit of the symptoms of a fallen arch usually lies in the improper function (locking and unlocking) of the foot during the gait cycle. This is discussed in more detail in Chapter 4.

A "fallen arch" is not a collapsed bridge!

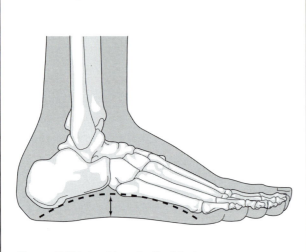

Figure 2-7 *Lateral Longitudinal Arch*

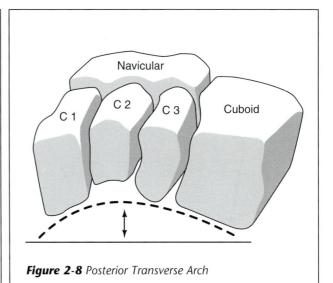

Figure 2-8 *Posterior Transverse Arch*

MUSCLES OF THE LOWER LEG

The muscles of the lower leg (Figure 2-9) govern the movements of the foot and are therefore included in the discussion of foot anatomy. Muscles allow us to move the specific parts of our bodies. They are attached at both ends (usually but not always) to bone. They are generally attached on either side of a joint. The *origin* of a muscle is the point where the muscle begins; it *inserts* by means of a tendon into the part that it is going to move. For purposes of this discussion rather than naming each individual muscle, its origin and insertion, we divide them into groups and discuss them in that manner.

——— L.O. 5

The lower leg muscles are divided into three groups—anterior, posterior, and lateral.

Anterior Extensor Group. This muscle group is composed of four muscles that pull the foot and toes up (extend or dorsiflex) toward the leg. One of these muscles inserts into the top of the big toe, another into the top of toes two through five, and one into the top of the foot itself. This muscle is the largest of the three and besides assisting in extension it also helps support the medial longitudinal arch. The last and smallest muscle of the group inserts into the top of the base and shaft of the fifth metatarsal.

Posterior Flexor Group. This group of muscles is divided into two layers, superficial and deep. Each layer has three muscles that extend into the foot. These muscles all help in pulling the foot and toes down (flex or plantarflex) away from the front of the leg.

The deep layer muscles insert one into the bottom of great toe, one into the bottom of toes two through five, and the other into the bottom middle of the foot where it also helps to support the medial longitudinal arch.

The superficial layer of muscles together form the calf of the leg and all end into the Achilles tendon that inserts into the heel bone or calcaneous. This tendon is the thickest and strongest tendon in the body.

Lateral Group. There are two muscles in this group. The larger one wraps its way under the middle of the foot where it inserts into the bottom of

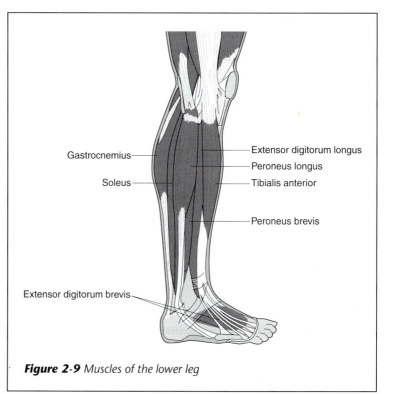

Gastrocnemius

Soleus

Extensor digitorum brevis

Extensor digitorum longus

Peroneus longus

Tibialis anterior

Peroneus brevis

Figure 2-9 *Muscles of the lower leg*

the first metatarsal cuneiform joint area where it helps to support the medial longitudinal arch as well as the posterior transverse arch. The other muscle inserts into the styloid process of the fifth metatarsal, helping to support the lateral longitudinal arch.

It is interesting how nature has allowed us to walk in the upright position. To lift our entire body weight, which is required of each foot during the gait cycle, we have six strong flexor muscles as compared to only three extensor muscles. Also the strongest, largest, and most durable tendon in our body is part of the flexor muscle group.

MUSCLES OF THE FOOT

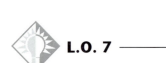

The bottom of the foot is more important than you might believe.

There are 20 small muscles in the foot of which 19 are located on the bottom of the foot. All of the muscles in the foot basically help to stabilize the toes during the gait cycle. When these muscles do not function properly during gait they help cause deformities such as hammertoes and bunions.

Dorsal Group

L.O. 6

The one muscle on the top of the foot is located on the lateral aspect just below the ankle. It may be visualized as a lump or mound of tissue in this area of the foot. This muscle is much more pronounced on some people than others. It helps to extend the toes as well as stabilize them during gait.

Plantar Groups

The plantar muscle groups can be divided into four distinct layers of muscle. The first layer is the most superficial (nearest the skin) and the fourth layer is the deepest, lying up next to the metatarsal bones.

L.O. 7

First Layer. The first layer of plantar muscles is composed of three muscles (Figure 2-10). The medial one goes to the big toe. The central muscle has four tendons that go to the second, third, fourth, and fifth toes. The lateral muscle inserts into the lateral side of the fifth toe.

Second Layer. This layer is composed of five muscles (Figure 2-11). These all basically help to stabilize and move the second, third, fourth, and fifth toes during gait.

Third Layer. There are four muscles in this layer (Figure 2-12). The most medial one inserts by two tendons into the sesamoid bones under the first metatarsal head and then on into the plantar aspect of the great toe. The two central muscles insert at an angle into the lateral sesamoid and then into the bottom of the great toe. These two muscles are really not necessary for proper function of the great toe. If we could use them as they were intended

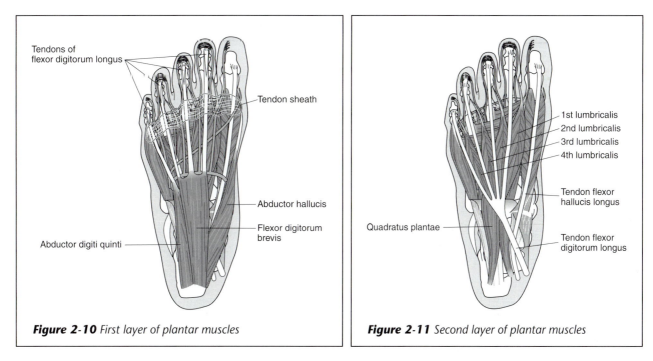

Figure 2-10 *First layer of plantar muscles*

Tendons of flexor digitorum longus

Tendon sheath

Abductor hallucis

Flexor digitorum brevis

Abductor digiti quinti

Figure 2-11 *Second layer of plantar muscles*

1st lumbricalis
2nd lumbricalis
3rd lumbricalis
4th lumbricalis

Tendon flexor hallucis longus

Quadratus plantae

Tendon flexor digitorum longus

we would have an opposable great toe that would work like our thumb so that we could grasp things. These muscles are really a big factor in helping to alter the position of the great toe during the development of a bunion deformity. The fourth muscle of this layer is on the lateral aspect of foot and inserts into the bottom of the proximal phalanx of the fifth toe.

Fourth Layer. This layer consists of seven very small muscles that are layered between the second, third, fourth, and fifth metatarsal shafts (Figure 2-13). They all insert into the bases of the proximal phalanges of the second, third, fourth, and fifth toes helping to stabilize them during gait.

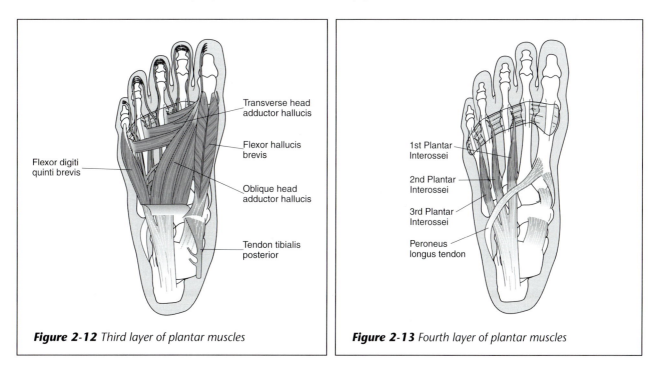

Figure 2-12 *Third layer of plantar muscles*

Transverse head adductor hallucis

Flexor hallucis brevis

Flexor digiti quinti brevis

Oblique head adductor hallucis

Tendon tibialis posterior

Figure 2-13 *Fourth layer of plantar muscles*

1st Plantar Interossei

2nd Plantar Interossei

3rd Plantar Interossei

Peroneus longus tendon

N E R V E S

Our nervous system and a house's electrical system are much the same!

You can compare the nervous system with the electrical wiring system of a house. Electricity passes through the wires to the lights, television, or other appliances of the house. Switches turn the electricity on and off to the different appliances or lights to make them work when they are needed. This is the same as the motor nervous system within our body. The brain tells the muscle to contract or relax by sending a stimulus through the nerve to tell the muscle to turn on or off. There is also a sensory nervous system part which allows us to feel touch, pressure, heat, cold, and pain. These are transmitted from nerve endings in the skin or other areas of the body. This system is also electrical but is more like the security alarm system in your house. Each room or area has sensors built into it to sense movement, vibrations, smoke, and so on. This is a simplistic explanation of how a very complex nervous system actually works. By simplifying it to this extent you will be able to visualize what is happening when we are walking or standing still.

L.O. 8 — The nerve supply to the foot arises from the spinal cord, in the sacral area of the low back, from a number of nerve roots. These unite to form the largest nerve in the body, the **sciatic nerve**. The sciatic nerve extends down the posterior aspect of the thigh to the knee. Here it divides into two branches, one going to the anterior aspect of the leg. This branch divides again and then both of these branches continue down the leg to the top of the foot. The second branch of the sciatic nerve continues down the posterior aspect of the leg where it enters the foot under the medial aspect of the ankle. It then branches again and continues branching until it reaches the ends of all the toes.

The sciatic nerve has both sensory and motor nerve fibers within it. As this nerve travels down the leg ending in the foot it gives off sensory branches to the skin and muscles while also giving off motor branches to the muscles. Changes in the low back that injure any one or all of the nerve roots that form the sciatic nerve can cause pain, or loss of sensation or movement in the leg or foot. This is only one reason that one must look at the entire person when treating or giving a service to the foot.

THE BLOOD SUPPLY—ARTERIES AND VEINS

The body's blood circulation functions much like the plumbing system in a house.

Blood is carried from the heart to the various parts of the body by **arteries**. If we continue comparisons, the arterial system is like the fresh water plumbing supply in a house. The water is brought into the house under pressure and shunted to the kitchen, bathrooms, and various other areas where it is needed.

The arteries are thick-walled elastic tubes or pipes. They are thick and elastic to withstand the pressure being exerted against them when the heart contracts. This is referred to as the **blood pressure**. Blood pressure is composed of the **systolic** and **diastolic** phases. The systolic phase is when the heart contracts and conversely the diastolic phase is when the heart relaxes. In measuring blood pressure what is really being measured is how much the artery expands and relaxes against a measured pressure being exerted against it by the blood pressure cuff (**sphygmomanometer**).

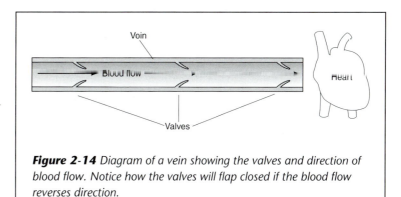

Figure 2-14 *Diagram of a vein showing the valves and direction of blood flow. Notice how the valves will flap closed if the blood flow reverses direction.*

Veins are thin-walled tubes or pipes. They could be loosely compared to the waste water plumbing system of a house. The water or waste in this system is not under pressure. Veins carry blood from the muscles and organs back to the heart. They are thin-walled because they do not have a lot of pressure being exerted against them when the heart contracts. Veins have many one-way valves (Figure 2-14) in them because of this. The valves allow the blood to flow only toward the heart. Many of the veins can be seen directly under the skin; arteries are usually deep under the tissues and we do not see them. Nature has done this as a protective mechanism. If an artery is cut a tremendous amount of blood may be lost in a very short time. They are therefore buried deep in the tissues as a protection. The large veins also are located along the large arteries for this same reason. In some areas on the body arteries are fairly superficial and can be seen expanding and contracting under the overlying tissue and skin. These are areas where the pulse rate is taken. When you **palpate** or "feel a pulse," you are feeling an artery expand and relax with each contraction and relaxation of the heart.

Blood reaches the foot by starting at the heart. From the heart, blood travels through the aorta, the largest artery of the body, to where it splits in the pelvis into the iliac arteries. These go into each thigh. From there it flows ——— **L.O. 9** into the femoral artery, a continuation of the iliac artery. The femoral artery becomes the popliteal artery in the lower third of the thigh. Just below the knee the popliteal artery divides into the anterior and posterior tibial arteries. The posterior tibial artery travels down the back of the leg entering the foot under the medial aspect of the ankle where it becomes the internal (medial) and external (lateral) plantar arteries. These arteries continue branching until they end in the plantar aspect of the toes. The anterior tibial artery passes,

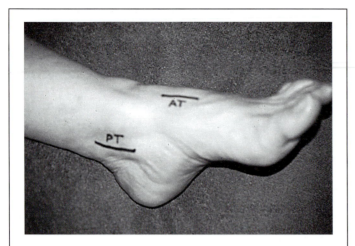

Figure 2-15 *The black line, AT, indicates the position of the dorsalis pedis pulse on the top of the foot. The black line, PT, indicates the position of the posterior tibial pulse on the medial side of the ankle.*

just below the knee, through the space between the leg bones (tibia and fibula) and extends down the front of the leg. At the anterior aspect of the ankle joint it becomes the dorsalis pedis artery. The dorsalis pedis artery lies over the talus, the navicular, and middle cuneiform bone. At this level it gives off branches that finally end in the top of the toes.

There are two places in the foot where a pulse may be felt. The first is on the top of the foot over the navicular and middle cuneiform bones. It is called the *dorsalis pedis pulse* because it is the dorsalis pedis artery that is being palpated. The second is palpated just below the **medial malleolus** of the tibia where the posterior tibial artery enters the foot. This pulse therefore is called the *posterior tibial pulse* (Figure 2-15).

This is a simple explanation of how a drop of blood travels from the heart to the end of the toes. What has to be remembered is that the main arteries are giving off branches to the various organs, muscles, bones, and skin as they pass these structures. These smaller arterial branches are called 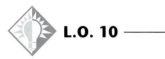 **arterioles**. The arterioles become **capillaries** in the structure to which the blood will supply oxygen and nutrients. Capillaries have a single cell wall that facilitates the passage of oxygen and other nutrients from the blood into the tissues. After passing through the tissues the capillaries become **venules** (small veins), which then become larger veins all ending back in the heart to start the process over.

BLOOD

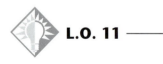 A discussion of the vascular system must be followed by a discussion of the elements flowing through this system. This is the blood (Figure 2-16). Blood is a very complex substance; however, for our purpose we will break it down into four basic parts.

1. **Plasma**—This is the fluid portion of the blood in which the solid parts are suspended. It composes 55% of the total volume of the blood. It is a clear straw-colored liquid, 92% water. The rest of its elements are plasma proteins, nutrients, gases, inorganic salts, various hormones, secretions, and enzymes.

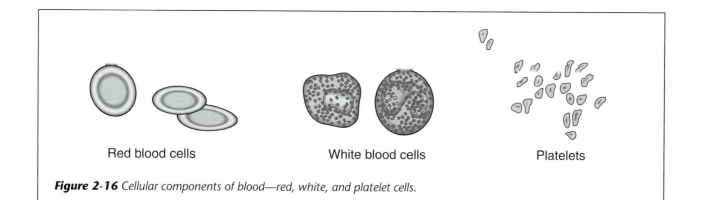

Red blood cells   White blood cells   Platelets

Figure 2-16 *Cellular components of blood—red, white, and platelet cells.*

2. **Erythrocytes** (red blood cells)—These cells transport oxygen to the tissues. **Hemoglobin** is the red part of the cell. Oxygen is attracted to the hemoglobin and attaches to it in the lungs. Oxygenated hemoglobin is then pumped into the heart and from there out into the arteries. Oxygenated blood is bright red in color and unoxygenated blood is darker red in color. This is the reason that arterial blood is bright red and venous blood is a darker red color.

3. **Leukocytes** (white blood cells)—These cells help protect the body from bacteria and other foreign bodies. They are able to travel through the walls of the blood vessels to the site of injury or infection. Here they are able to engulf (**phagocytize**) the bacteria or foreign body and destroy it. **Pus** is mainly composed of dead white blood cells that have died after doing their job.

4. **Thrombocytes** (platelets)—These are the main clotting elements within the blood. They have the capability of adhering to uneven or damaged surfaces forming a foundation to which the other clotting elements of the blood adhere. This then is the blood clot that is the beginning of the healing process after an injury.

LYMPHATIC SYSTEM

As the blood travels through the capillaries, the fluid portion of plasma is transferred through the capillary walls into the tissue spaces. Once the plasma leaves the blood vascular system and enters the tissue spaces it is called **lymphatic** fluid or **lymph**. These spaces within the tissues allow the tissue fluid or lymphatic fluid to come into contact with the individual cells of the tissues themselves. (Remember the tissue fluids contain many things necessary for cell life and growth such as nutrients from the stomach and small intestine.) These tissue spaces are the beginning of the lymphatic system.

—— **L.O. 12**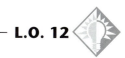

The lymphatic system is a vast, complex network of capillaries, thin vessels, valves, ducts, nodes, and organs. They help to maintain the internal fluid environment of the entire body by producing, filtering, and conveying lymph from the tissues back into the blood vascular system of the body. The white blood cells travel freely from the vascular system into the lymphatic system to function at sites of injury and infection. Some white cells are actually formed within the lymphatic system. The so-called red streak often seen extending from the site of an infection in the foot or other area of the body is actually an inflammation of a lymphatic vessel (**lymphangitis**). Along with this condition, swollen tender lymph nodes are usually also found behind the knee or in the groin areas if the infection is in the foot or leg. If this condition is observed, it is imperative the individual see a doctor for treatment of the infection. Any delay will let the infection spread into other areas of the body possibly with disastrous consequences.

An infection's red streak is actually an inflamed lymph vessel.

The lymphatic capillaries, which connect the tissue spaces to the lymphatic vessels, start in the skin and form a continuous network over and through the entire body. There is no pressure to move the lymph through the system except that pressure exerted from the surrounding areas of the body, such as muscle contractions or gravity. The lymphatic vessels have valves in them similar to the valves seen in the veins. These prevent the backflow of the lymphatic fluid in the system. If the valves do not function or the system has a blockage in it we then see swelling of the tissues. This is called **edema** or excess fluid in the tissue spaces. The foot and leg are particularly susceptible to this condition because of their distant position from the heart. In these areas, gravity and **hydrostatic** pressure are working against the lymphatic system and compound the problem of swelling in the lower extremity.

It is important to understand the lymphatic system. When giving a massage of the foot and leg one is promoting the flow of lymphatic fluid from the foot, ankle, and leg back into the general lymphatic system. This helps to relieve pressure and congestion and gives a feeling of well-being and relaxation. It also promotes a healthier environment for the structures of the foot and leg to function. It is important that one develop a good technique when giving a foot and leg massage.

SKIN OR INTEGUMENTARY SYSTEM

The skin is the outermost covering of the body and is the organ system that the beauty professional is actually working on. Most products within the industry have some direct or indirect effect on the skin. The cosmetic appearance of this body covering is of great importance to the individual. Practices such as scarring, branding, piercing, and tattooing all permanently change the structure and appearance of the skin in the name of beauty. Powders, creams, oils, and paints applied to its surface temporarily change its appearance, again in the name of beauty. It is imperative that a full knowledge of this system be obtained before performing any service on it. That is why this section will go into more detail than the previous anatomic discussions.

Skin comprises the largest organ system of the body. The skin of an average-sized man is estimated to weigh approximately 10 pounds and 7 pounds for the average woman. It covers an area of about 15,000 square inches, which is almost the size of a 9' x 12' rug. It is the most visible portion of our entire anatomy.

The skin performs many vital functions necessary for life. It forms a protective barrier against injury and infections to the underlying tissues. The formation of a **callous** in areas of pressure or friction is one of its protective functions. It helps to insulate the body from heat and cold. It helps control body temperature by the formation of perspiration that evaporates, thus assisting in cooling the body. Perspiration also helps to eliminate some body wastes. If allowed to build up on the skin, these wastes can cause an offensive odor. It guards against excessive exposure to ultraviolet (UV) light by the production of pigments as well as using this same UV light to produce the body's supply of vitamin D. It allows us to be in contact with our surroundings through the sensory receptors for pain, touch, pressure, cold, and heat contained within it.

In the feet and hands, as in no other places in the body, are its functions of protection and sensations of touch, pressure, pain, hot, and cold more important. These two areas of our body are in almost constant direct contact with our surroundings. They are extremely dependent on the skin and its sensory organs for information allowing us to live and work safely in our environment.

The skin is divided into three layers: **epidermis** (outermost layer), **dermis** also known as corium, and the **hypodermis** (fatty or innermost layer) (Figure 2-17).

The largest organ in the body weighs between 7 and 10 pounds and has several important functions.

——— **L.O. 13**

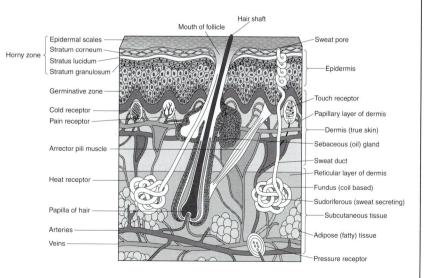

Figure 2-17 *Cross-section of the skin*

Labels in figure: Hair shaft, Mouth of follicle, Sweat pore, Epidermal scales, Stratum corneum, Stratus lucidum, Stratum granulosum, Horny zone, Germinative zone, Cold receptor, Pain receptor, Arrector pili muscle, Heat receptor, Papilla of hair, Arteries, Veins, Epidermis, Touch receptor, Papillary layer of dermis, Dermis (true skin), Sebaceous (oil) gland, Sweat duct, Reticular layer of dermis, Fundus (coil based), Sudoriferous (sweat secreting), Subcutaneous tissue, Adipose (fatty) tissue, Pressure receptor

Epidermis

The epidermis on most of the body is about the thickness of a sheet of paper (approximately 0.2 mm). On the soles of the feet and palms of the hands it is much thicker. The extra thickness in these areas is not due primarily to pressure or friction. This is shown to be true by the fact that if skin from the sole or palm is grafted to another area of the body it continues to have the same thickness and appearance. There are no blood vessels or lymph channels in the epidermis; it must depend on tissue fluid for its nutrition. It contains free ends of nerves that transmit pain sensations. **Melanocytes** or pigment cells are also contained within the epidermis. It is attached to the underlying layer by tissue extensions coming up into it from the dermis.

Your epidermis is showing!

Microscopically, the epidermis is composed of five distinct layers, each one giving rise to the next layer of cells. The estimated time it takes for cells to progress from the basal layer to the horny or outer layer is 28 days. This process is called **keratinization.**

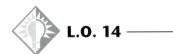 **L.O. 14**

1. **Basal cell layer**—One cell layer in thickness and gives rise to all of the cells in the other four layers.

2. **Prickle cell layer** (stratum spinosum, or malpighian layer)—Is in most cases the thickest cell layer of the epidermis. The cells of this layer are separated by small spaces much like the tissue spaces. The cells of this layer are connected together by small intercellular bridges or prickles extending from cell to cell through the spaces. These cell spaces probably are important in the nutrition and metabolic exchanges of the cells.

3. **Granular cell layer** (stratum granulosum)—The thickness of this layer varies from one to three cell layers. It is thickest in areas where there is callus formation. The intercellular bridges of the prickle cell layer have all but vanished.

4. **Clear cell layer** (stratum lucidum)—A narrow band of flattened cells that have no nuclei within them. This makes them appear clear when viewed under the microscope. This layer is visible mainly in the epidermis of the soles of the feet and the palms of the hands.

5. **Horny cell layer** (stratum corneum)—Outer layer of the skin, composed of dead cells and varying in thickness depending on the area in which it lies. The thickest areas are on the soles and palms. This layer is constantly being worn away by normal daily living activities. The estimated daily loss is between 0.5 and 1 gram. It is noteworthy that in a condition called exfoliative dermatitis the daily loss of this layer may reach 9 to 17 grams.

Dermis

The dermis or corium is the next main layer of the skin. It is the layer to which the epidermis attaches. It makes up 15% to 20% of total body weight. This layer is thicker on the soles and palms. The main elements found in the dermis are **collagen** and elastin that form the elastic fibers found here. Collagen makes up 95% of the mass of the dermis. The elastic fibers in this layer give stretch and resilience to the skin.

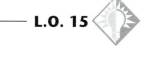 L.O. 15

Microscopically the dermis is divided into two layers.

1. **Stratum papillare**—This layer consists of finger-like projections, called papillare or papillary bodies, which extend up into the epidermis. They give a large surface area for attachment of the epidermis to the underlying dermis.

2. **Stratum reticulare**—This layer is directly under the papillary layer.

These two layers cannot be clearly separated. In the reticulare layer the collagen fibers are densely packed and run more or less parallel to the surface of the skin. The collagen fibers in the papillare layer are much thinner and loosely arranged. The collagen fibers in both layers are arranged into bundles that are then connected to one another by the elastic fibers found within the dermis. Throughout the dermis is a vast network of capillaries, both vascular and lymphatic, as well as nerves and nerve endings.

Hypodermis

The hypodermis or subcutaneous layer of the skin is in part a continuation of the dermis. Its collagen and elastic fibers are not as dense as in the dermis. These fibers run into the dermis and connect it to the underlying tissues. Where the skin is flexible the fibers in this layer are few. Where it is closely attached to the underlying parts, as in the soles and palms, the fibers are thick and numerous.

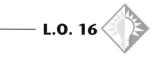 L.O. 16

Within the hypodermis, depending on the area of the body, there are varying numbers of fat cells. These cells make up the bulk of this subcutaneous layer. Also found within the hypodermis are many large blood vessels, nerves, lymph vessels, and nerve endings.

SKIN APPENDAGES

The epidermis in many areas folds in down into the dermis where it becomes modified to form different structures and appendages. These include hair, nails, sweat glands, and sebaceous glands.

L.O. 17

Hair

Hair is distributed in varying density and types over the body. No hair follicles are found on the sides and bottoms of the toes, the soles, and the side surfaces below the ankle.

Nails

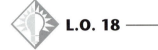
L.O. 18

Nails are horny plates on the dorsal surface of the distal phalanges of the toes and fingers. The surface of the skin covered by them is the **nail bed**. The surface of the nail bed is the malpighian or prickle cell layer of the epidermis. The nail bed and nail are surrounded laterally and proximally by a fold of skin called the *nail wall*. The slit between the wall and the bed is called the *nail groove*. As the skin turns into the groove it loses its horny, clear, and granular layers. Thus the nail bed as stated is only composed of the hypodermis, dermis, and the basal and prickle cell layers of the epidermis. Under the proximal fold the horny, clear, and granular layers end on the top of the nail as the **eponychium**. Under the distal or free edge of the nail the same thing happens with the epidermis and here it is called the **hyponychium**. The base or root of the nail has a whitish semilunar area that is called the **lunula**. The lunula is the visible portion of the **matrix bed**. It is from the matrix bed that the formation of nail substance proceeds. As new nail is formed in the matrix bed the older portions of the nail move distally over the rest of the nail bed. Most experts believe that only the matrix portion of the nail bed actually forms nail substance. They seem to agree that once formed the nail plate simply glides over the the nail bed.

Sweat Glands

Sweat glands, more particularly eccrine sweat glands, are located throughout most areas of the skin. They are simple coiled tubular glands extending down from the epidermis into the dermis. They are most concentrated in the soles, palms, and axilla (armpit) areas of the body. The eccrine sweat glands are the only skin appendages on the soles of the feet. These glands produce sweat to help control body temperatures.

Sebaceous Glands

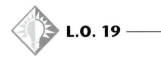
L.O. 19

Sebaceous glands are scattered over the surface of the skin where there is hair growth. These glands are located in the dermis from extensions of the epidermis. They open into the necks of the hair follicles. They produce sebum, which is a lipid-rich substance that helps to keep the skin and hair from drying out. Because there is very little hair growth in the feet there are also few sebaceous glands present. Because of this the use of moisturizer preparations on the feet is particularly essential.

FOOT NOTES

This chapter is the building block on which to build the rest of your knowledge of the maintence and care of the human foot. Anatomy is the basis for any study of the human body. An understanding of basic anatomy is essential. Without it you will be working in the dark when giving clients a nail or foot service. Use this chapter as a reference as you read other chapters of this book.

QUESTIONS

1. What is the largest bone in the foot?

2. How many muscles originate and insert only in the foot?

3. Name the two places on the foot where the pulse may be taken.

4. What structure are you observing when you see a "red streak" extending up the leg from an infected big toe?

5. What is edema?

6. What is the largest organ system of the body?

7. What makes up almost 95% of the mass of the skin layer called the dermis?

8. Name the four different skin appendages.

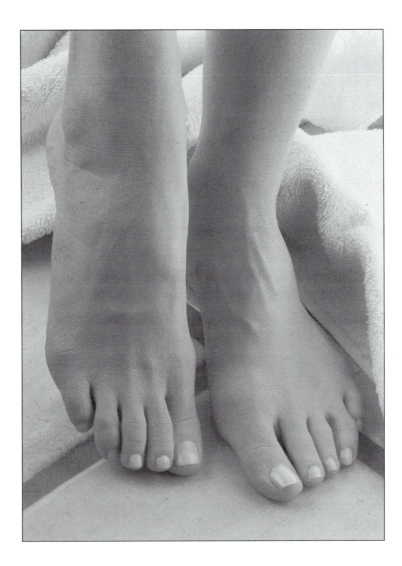

Systemic Diseases and the Foot

3

LEARNING OBJECTIVES

After studying this chapter, the reader should be able to:

1. Discuss how abuse of alcohol, drugs, and nicotine affect the foot.

2. Define scleroderma and describe its effect on the skin and feet.

3. Compare and contrast Raynaud's disease and phenomenon.

4. Outline the characteristics of inflammatory and noninflammatory arthritis.

5. Describe the features of rheumatoid arthritis.

6. Describe the features of gout.

7. Compare primary and secondary osteoarthritis.

8. Describe the effects of congestive heart disease and pulmonary hypertension on the lower leg.

9. Describe the signs of subacute bacterial endocarditis.

10. Describe the signs of anemia seen in the feet.

11. Outline the type of care offered to a client who has had a cerebrovascular accident.

12. Discuss the forms, development, and signs and symptoms of arteriosclerosis obliterans.

13. Identify the causes of diabetes.

14. Differentiate betweeen type 1 and type 2 diabetes mellitus.

15. Briefly describe the oral glucose tolerance test procedure.

16. Describe the effects of diabetes on the skin, vascular system, nerves, and feet.

17. Outline the questions that should be asked of clients who are diabetic.

The condition of the foot may indicate the presence of a systemic disease.

This chapter discusses **systemic** (affecting the entire body) diseases that may be recognized by signs or symptoms seen in the foot. Systemic diseases such as diabetes affect the entire body. In these cases it is imperative that the whole client be evaluated. Remember that the foot comes with a human being attached to it. By being able to see the changes in the foot associated with certain diseases you will be able to render and recommend safe pedicure services for the client. You will also be better prepared to discuss your client's care with a medical professional should the occasion require.

ABUSIVE DISEASES

These diseases involve the overuse of chemical substances that result in harm being caused to the individual who is abusing the substance. Those who may be in direct or indirect contact with that individual may also suffer harm as the result of the chemical abuse. Alcohol, drugs (legal or illegal, prescription or over-the-counter), nicotine in the form of smoking, and inhalants such as paint or glue fumes all may be classified as chemicals with a potential for abuse. For the purposes of this text the discussion will be confined to the health aspects of this abuse and how its secondary effects may relate to the foot.

Alcohol

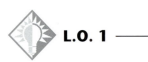

L.O. 1

Excessive use of alcohol may affect the ability to heal. It may also cause liver disease, kidney disease, **gout**, and **anemias**. In the foot, swelling caused by these conditions may be the only sign that may lead to a suspicion that a problem exists. Another thing seen in an alcoholic is a general disregard for personal hygiene. The foot in particular shows this by a general buildup of dead skin and debris between the toes. The nails are usually dirty, unkempt, thick, and discolored. A good pedicure will help this individual prevent foot infections and will make him or her feel better in general. WARNING: Be careful not to cut the client when trimming the nails. These individuals are more prone to infection and do not heal well.

Drugs (Legal or Illegal)

Legal prescription drugs, some over-the-counter drugs, and illegal drugs may cause conditions similar to those seen in alcohol abuse. Always evaluate the entire individual. If there is any question in your mind about recommending a service do not do it! Care must be taken to recommend and give services that will not cause harm.

Nicotine (Smoking)

Heavy smoking causes lung disease, and generalized vascular changes. Nicotine is a poison and has a cumulative affect on the tissues. **Emphysema**, hardening of the arteries, and vasospastic diseases may all be caused or made worse by smoking. You can usually tell a long-time smoker by looking at the skin of the feet. The changes are subtle but are evident if you look for them. The skin is thin and translucent, loses its elasticity, and looks totally different from normal healthy skin. These changes are particularly evident around the nails and in the toes. If you have done the history and personal examination and basically find a healthy client but still see changes in the skin that do not appear normal ask if the client smokes. The answer is usually yes! A pedicure is a safe procedure with these clients. Be careful not to cut them when trimming the nails because they usually are slow to heal.

Buerger's disease (thromboangiitis obliterans) is directly related to smoking. It is most often seen in men between the ages of 20 to 40. It is rarely seen in women. The nicotine from the cigarette causes the platelets (those primary cells within the blood that help with blood clotting) to become more adhesive. This results in clot formation within the intermediate small-sized arteries and veins of the extremities. **Intermittent claudication**, which is a condition in which exercise causes the muscles of the leg to cramp and become painful because of lack of oxygen, is one of the first complaints of Buerger's disease. The client will tell you that he can only walk so far, half a block, a block, before he must stop and rest for a few minutes before continuing on. As it progresses and more and larger clots are formed within the vessels, gangrenous changes in the tips of the digits may be noted. Treatment to restore the circulation will not help until the individual has stopped smoking.

A client with Buerger's disease should be referred to the podiatrist for general foot and nail care.

The skin appearance will be the same as that seen in severe cases of hardening of the arteries (see later in this chapter). It will be thin and dry, and the tissues will lose their elasticity. **Cyanosis** may be present in those areas most affected by the loss of circulation. As the disease progresses patches of **gangrene** occur due to this loss of circulation. Remember to listen to the client history for complaints of intermittent claudication, which may be the first symptom of this disease. A client with Buerger's disease should be referred to the podiatrist for general foot and nail care. A podiatrist will be able to recognize early changes, and the client should then be referred for more intensive medical care. These clients should not receive foot services from the nail professional.

These are diseases resulting from the **immune** system identifying tissues within the body as being foreign. In most instances the cause of the disease process is unknown. A few of them that can affect how pedicure services are rendered are discussed here.

Scleroderma (Progressive Systemic Sclerosis)

L.O. 2

This is a disease of unknown **etiology** causing sclerosis (hardening) of the connective tissues within the body. Excessive **collagen** is deposited within these tissues. Women are affected two to three times more frequently than men. The esophagus, intestines, heart, lungs, and kidneys may be affected. The skin in particular is affected, thus the name scleroderma (hard skin). The large amount of collagen deposited within the skin causes it to lose its elasticity and stretching abilities. The small vessels within the skin are also affected and become blocked.

Changes in the nails may be a clue to scleroderma.

Changes seen within the feet often lead to the final diagnosis of this condition. The skin of the feet becomes shiny, smooth, and thickened. The nails in clients with long-standing disease may have longitudinal ridges extending from the base of the nail to the free edge. They also become thinned to the point they split along these ridges. Because of the thinning the nail bed causes the nail to have a red hue. Other nail changes seen may be **pterygium** formation where normal skin overgrows and fuses to the nail plate. Beau's lines (transverse grooves) across the nail may also be seen. Small painful ulcers may form on the toes because of the vascular changes in the small blood vessels of the skin. When these heal they will leave a small indentation in the skin.

Most of these clients will already be aware of their disease before seeking a pedicure. If open ulcerations are present the client should be referred for medical care; otherwise a pedicure is not contraindicated. The main thing to remember is to be very gentle with the service. Hydrating creams and cuticle oils should be recommended to help the skin.

Raynaud's Syndrome

This is a condition in which the small arteries in the feet and hands go into vasospasm (constrict) in response to cold temperatures or emotional factors. This causes the affected tissues or digits to appear white or bluish (cyanotic) because of the decreased blood supply to the tissues. The mere act of reaching into the freezer to get something can trigger the vasospasm. When the spasm abates the tissues or digits tingle, become red, and throb. The client may complain of **chronic** coldness in the hands and feet. The fingers may remain bluish and cold while the feet, because they are protected by hosiery and footwear, may not be as affected.

— L.O. 3

This **syndrome** can be divided into two distinct entities—Raynaud's disease and Raynaud's phenomenon. The actual cause of Raynaud's disease is unknown. It is most commonly seen in women between the ages of 20 and 40. It has a gradual onset. Early symptoms may be a mild short-lasting attack in the winter. In the later stages the attacks last longer, nails grow more slowly and become brittle and deformed. Raynaud's phenomenon is seen secondary to diseases such as Buerger's disease, vascular injuries, hardening of the arteries (arteriosclerosis obliterans), **neurogenic** disorders, exposure to certain chemicals, and connective tissue diseases such as scleroderma.

The nail professional needs to determine the severity of the syndrome before administering a service. In the later stages the slightest break in the skin can cause an ulceration that is easily infected and takes a long time to heal. A referral to the podiatrist for routine foot care is the proper way of handling the client with late stage disease. If the syndrome is in its early stages a pedicure by the nail professional is not contraindicated. Be gentle and recommend products that will assist in maintaining a healthy skin.

Acrocyanosis

This condition also causes a spasm of the superficial arterioles secondary to cold exposure with a resultant cyanotic appearance of the skin. It is a **benign** condition (one that causes no harm) that does not need treatment. It is seen more often in women and affects both the hands and feet. There are no symptoms associated with it other than the cyanosis. The color changes generally affect the whole hand or foot and may even extend up the arm or leg. In Raynaud's the digits are usually the only affected areas. The skin of the palms of the hands is usually wet and clammy in acrocyanosis, whereas in Raynaud's it is dry.

Pedicure services may be safely given to these individuals. The main thing to do before the service is to know the difference between acrocyanosis and Raynaud's disease. If there is any question about the client's condition talk to the client's physician or podiatrist before performing the service.

You must know the difference between acrocyanosis and Raynaud's disease.

A R T H R I T I D E S

This section discusses the various forms of arthritis the nail professional should be aware of. **Arthritis** is defined as a condition that causes swelling of a joint with resulting pain. Different types of arthritis affect different parts

— L.O. 4

of the joints. By eliciting proper information from the client you will be able to generally determine what type of arthritis is present.

Arthritis is divided into two types: inflammatory and noninflammatory. The basic characteristics of the two types are listed in Table 3-1.

Table 3-1 Characteristics of Inflammatory and Noninflammatory Arthritis

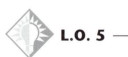
L.O. 4

Inflammatory	Noninflammatory
Bone destroyed	New bone formed
Long periods of stiffness after rest	Short periods of stiffness after rest
Pain at rest	Minimal or no pain at rest
Hot, red swollen joints	Minimal heat or color changes around affected joints
May have fevers, weight loss, skin rashes, loss of appetite	Usually no systemic symptoms

Inflammatory Types of Arthritis

L.O. 5

Rheumatoid Arthritis. This is a chronic systemic type of arthritis involving mainly the small joints of the hands and feet (Figure 3-1). The synovial lining or membrane of the joint capsule is the portion of the joint initially affected. The soft tissues around the joints become swollen, red, and warm. Later changes result in *bone and articular surface destruction* with resultant abnormalities. The cause is not known. It is seen more commonly in women than men, a 3:1 ratio. It can be seen in any age group but the peak age of onset is from 25 to 50. The most common onset is gradual, involving numerous small joints of the hands and feet with resultant stiffness and generalized fatigue. Other joints are affected as the disease progresses. Both feet are usually affected with the metatarsophalangeal joints most commonly being involved.

As the disease progresses gross deformities are seen in the finger and toe joints. The digits deviate away from the midline of the body. **Hammertoes** and **bunions** develop. The fat pad under the ball of the foot thins and the metatarsal heads are easily felt (palpated).

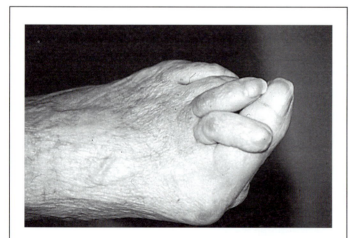

Figure 3-1 *Rheumatoid arthritis in the feet. Notice the severe deformities and dislocations in the toes at the metatarsal phalangeal joints.*

Pressure ulcers may form in these areas as a result of this thinning. Small cysts called rheumatoid nodules form under the skin in areas of pressure. These may also rupture and ulcerate through the skin.

As a general statement rheumatoid individuals are irritable and have a very low pain threshold. This is the result of being in pain most of the time. They lose sleep because of this and are constantly reminded of their disease. In the absence of open ulcerations and infection, it is safe to give these clients a pedicure service. A warm hydrotherapy bath for the feet and possibly even a hot wax service will give short-term symptomatic relief and will be a pleasure for the client. Be gentle in the massage and nail portion of the pedicure. These clients will not tolerate any added discomfort.

Psoriatic Arthritis. Six percent of individuals with psoriasis (to be discussed later under skin diseases) will develop an inflammatory arthritis. The most common indication of this process is a "sausage digit." This is a diffuse swelling of toes. In most instances pain is associated with this condition. The distal and intermediate phalangeal joints are most frequently involved with psoriatic arthritis. Typical "punched out" areas of *bone destruction* are seen in these areas.

In the absence of open **lesions** a pedicure service may be safely performed on these clients. As with other arthritic conditions the service must be gentle.

Gout. This disease affects approximately 3% of the population. It affects men in the majority of the cases. Only 5% of those who have gout are women. It is not a disease of the rich and may be seen in all socioeconomic levels of society. The two types of gout are primary and secondary.

—— **L.O. 6**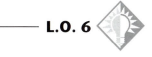

> *Gout is most often he result of improper elimination of uric acid from the body.*

- *Primary gout* is an inherited disorder of uric acid metabolism. Usually the kidney is not excreting the uric acid properly.

- *Secondary gout* is caused by the overproduction of uric acid by certain types of cancers, psoriasis, obesity, over ingestion of alcohol, and some types of anemias. Secondary gout can also be caused by **diuretic** medications (water pills), which cause an underexcretion of uric acid.

Gout is most often the result of improper elimination of uric acid from the body. It may also be caused by an overproduction of uric acid that then cannot be eliminated by the kidney fast enough. Because uric acid is not readily **soluble** in fluids, it **precipitates** out of solution in the form of urate crystals. The first metatarsophalangeal joint (great toe joint) is the usual site involved in a gouty attack. When this joint is involved it is classically called "podagra." The joint and surrounding tissues become acutely painful and swollen and have a deep reddish color. Other joints of the foot may be affected including those of the midtarsal area as well as the ankle. Other joints in the body may also be affected but those of the foot remain the most commonly involved.

Clients never think they have gout—they know it! The pain is extreme, coming on very rapidly, usually at night, and is not relieved by changing positions, soaking, or taking over-the-counter pain medications. The crystal deposits (**tophi**) of uric acid act as an extreme irritant to the joint and surrounding soft tissues, thus causing the acute unrelenting pain.

After the acute attack has subsided a chronic inflammatory arthritis of the involved joint may occur. This is caused by leftover deposits of the urate crystals within the joint that are imbedded within the joint cartilage. The uric acid destroys the cartilage, resulting in the actual arthritic changes that cause swelling and pain of the joint. Uric acid deposits may also remain in the soft tissues and ulcerate through the skin. A white paste-like drainage can be seen, which is the actual uric acid crystals.

A foot service may be performed as long as no open ulcers are present. If a client with an **acute** attack should happen to ask for a foot service, which is doubtful, he or she should be immediately referred to a physician or podiatrist for care. With proper medication, usually Indocin, an acute attack can be dramatically relieved.

Noninflammatory Arthritis

Osteoarthritis. This is the most common type of arthritis. Seventy-five to 80% of the population over 65 years of age suffer from at least a mild form of osteoarthritis.

L.O. 7

The two types of osteoarthritis are primary and secondary. *Primary osteoarthritis* is more common in women and 60% of those who have it show a positive family history of the disease. The early disease process of the primary type involves mainly the proximal and distal interphalangeal joints of the hands. *Secondary osteoarthritis* is the most common type and is caused by wear and tear on the joints. The weight-bearing joints of the body are subjected to extra stress and wear and are the main joints involved in the secondary form. The thumb joint (first carpometacarpal joint) is often the first joint affected in women. Certain types of jobs put extra stress on particular joints causing excessive wear. Ballet dancers put extra stress on the ankle joints that then become osteoarthritic; under normal circumstances the ankle joint is rarely involved in this disease process. Malpositioning of a joint, such as in a bunion deformity of the great toe joint (Figure 3-2), causes abnormal wear resulting in osteoarthritic changes in and around the joint.

Osteoarthritis starts with a breakdown of the cartilage within the joint. This results in bone rubbing on bone causing further injury within the joint. New bone is formed in the body's attempt to repair the damage. This new bone growth is seen as bony spurring around the joints. A bunion is a form of new bone growth as are the bony bumps seen on the fingers of the elderly. This new bone formation is just the opposite of the inflammatory types of arthritis in which bone is destroyed. This, therefore, is one way of differentiating between inflammatory and noninflammatory types of arthritis.

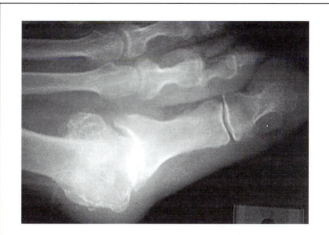

Figure 3-2 *An x-ray of osteoarthritis of the first metatarsal phalangeal joint. There is new bone formation around the metatarsal head (the bunion) and spurring on the base of the proximal phalanx.*

Swollen joints, mainly from the extra bone formation, mild morning stiffness, and the absence of heat or redness are all typical symptoms of this process. Weather changes can also cause pain and stiffness in the osteoarthritic joints. Who has not heard someone say "a storm must be coming because my arthritis is acting up!" Loss of motion within the joint is progressive with the loss of cartilage. In the foot, bunions, hammertoes, and **bone spurs (exostosis)**, are a common result of this disease.

A pedicure service will be appreciated by clients with osteoarthritis. Warmth and a gentle massage will give temporary relief to symptoms. They will also appreciate the nail care because in most instances they have a hard time reaching their feet because of stiffness and pain in their knees, hips, or back. A proper foot service will make them a long-term satisfied client.

Traumatic Arthritis. Traumatic arthritis is the result of injury to a joint, and thus, may be classified as a secondary form of osteoarthritis. It is basically the same as osteoarthritis in that the body tries to repair itself by the formation of new bone at the injured sight. The injury caused a break in the cartilage and from there on the process is the same as osteoarthritis. Foot services have the same indications as in the osteoarthritic client.

CARDIOVASCULAR DISEASE

These are diseases that affect the heart with secondary effects on surrounding organs and areas of the body away from the heart.

Congestive Heart Disease

This condition is caused by the failure of the heart to pump enough blood. This then results in back-pressure on the vascular system, which causes excessive swelling (edema) in the feet and legs. This swelling does not go down at

Back-pressure on the vascular system causes excessive swelling (edema) in the feet and legs.

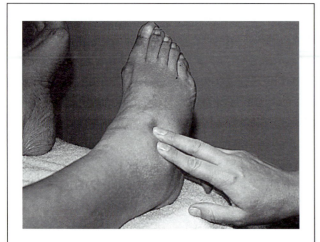

Figure 3-3 *To demonstrate pitting edema pressure is firmly applied to the swollen area with the fingers.*

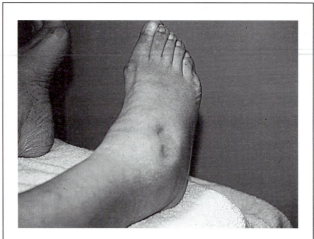

Figure 3-4 *Upon releasing the pressure a pit or depression is left because the fluid has been compressed out of the underlying tissues. As the fluid is replaced the pit gradually disappears. This picture would represent a 4+ pitting edema.*

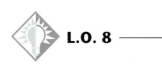

L.O. 8

night or when the extremity is elevated. Pitting edema (Figures 3-3 and 3-4) is present in varying degrees depending on the severity of the heart failure. The edema may become so severe that the tissues will not compress, or "pit," and they become almost rock hard. If this condition is present one may observe small droplets of fluid on the skin surface of the lower leg. This is tissue fluid that has been forced through the skin because of the extreme back-pressure on the vascular system. Open ulcers (stasis ulcers) may form in the lower leg and foot from pressure and lack of adequate **oxygenation** to the skin and underlying tissues. The skin in the leg and foot may become red and irritated in a condition known as **stasis dermatitis**.

Any type of physical activity in these individuals causes shortness of breath. The more severe the condition the harder it is for the individual to breathe. The condition can come on very slowly and patients do not realize what is happening or that they are experiencing a heart problem. They will come in for their routine foot care and need referral to their primary care physician or cardiologist for medical care. If someone like this comes into your salon you will be doing a favor to suggest that he or she see a physician.

As long as there are no open ulcers a foot service is not contraindicated in the milder forms of congestive heart failure. The service may also be performed on individuals who are already receiving medical care for the condition. If you question whether or not to provide the service contact the client's physician before proceeding. By being able to recognize the condition you will be better able to serve your clients in a more professional manner.

Heart disease can have devastating effects on the lower legs and feet.

Pulmonary Hypertension

This is a condition caused by excessive back-pressure within the arterial supply of the lungs. The most common cause of this is emphysema associated with long-term smoking. Surgical removal of a lung, injuries to the chest, and blood clots in the lung are less common causes.

This condition is mentioned because the lower extremity symptoms mimic those seen in congestive heart disease. Foot services in these individuals should be approached in a similar manner as in those clients with congestive heart disease.

Subacute Bacterial Endocarditis

Subacute bacterial endocarditis (SBE) is a bacterial infection affecting the inner lining of the heart. The subacute form does not cause heart symptoms. General symptoms such as **malaise** (a vague feeling of bodily discomfort), chills, and fever may be present. Small blood clots (emboli) may form on the infected lining of the heart. These may be dislodged and expelled into the vascular system. If these emboli lodge in the small arteries in the lungs a condition called embolic pneumonia may result.

Clubbing of the toes (more commonly seen in the fingers), splinter hemorrhages (small black lines), or **petechiae** (small red or purplish spots) in the nails, Janeway lesions (hemorrhagic spots) on the soles and palms, and Osler's nodes (small red-purple raised lesion that may or may not have a white center at the ends of the toes or fingers) may be seen as signs of SBE in the extremities.

——— L.O. 9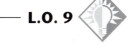

By knowing the signs of SBE you may be able to direct these clients to their physician for an evaluation. With some of the primary visual signs of this disease being seen in the hands and feet you may be the first to recognize them. A foot service is not contraindicated in a client with SBE as long as the person is aware he has the condition. If he is unaware of it, you should refer the client to the physician for evaluation before rendering the service.

ANEMIA

Anemia is a reduction of the **hemoglobin** level within the red blood cells, which results in a decrease in the oxygen-carrying capacity of the blood. Hemoglobin, which is the oxygen-carrying component of the blood, is the red portion of the red blood cell. Anemia can be caused by the chronic loss of blood (as in a long-term bleeding ulcer of the stomach or bowel), excessive destruction of the red blood cells by certain poisons, or immune system disorders such as sickle cell anemia, and in infections such as malaria. Another cause of anemia is a disease named pernicious anemia, which is caused by an

Anemia is a reduction of the hemoglobin level within the red blood cells.

inability to absorb vitamin B12 in the intestinal tract. Because of the lack of vitamin B12, the body is unable to produce red blood cells or hemoglobin and the individual becomes gradually more anemic.

Signs of anemias seen in the feet and hands may be numbness, tingling, or nerve pain (**neuralgia**). Numbness is often the first symptom seen in the feet and hands of individuals with pernicious anemia. The nails may become excessively brittle, spoon shaped, flat, or concave. Edema of the feet and ankles is often seen in individuals with anemia. Severely anemic individuals may exhibit mental confusion, and their coloring appears pasty and blanched out.

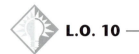 **L.O. 10**

It is all right to give foot services to clients with anemia as long as they are under a doctor's care for the condition. WARNING: Be gentle and do not use excessively hot water for the foot soak. By knowing the signs and symptoms of this condition you will be better prepared to service an anemic client. You may even be the first one to see a client whom you may suspect has an anemia and be able to refer him or her to a doctor for an evaluation.

CEREBROVASCULAR ACCIDENT

The death of the brain cells causes many devastating physical problems.

A cerebrovascular accident (CVA) or stroke is the destruction of brain cells as the result of a loss of oxygen to those cells. This can be caused by a ruptured blood vessel, a blocked blood vessel, or even a decreased flow of blood that does not allow sufficient oxygen to the tissues of the brain. Depending on the area, the death of the brain cells causes many devastating physical problems.

In the lower extremity and foot a stroke can cause many different signs and symptoms. Loss of feeling, **spasticity**, **paralysis**, muscle contractures, and swelling are all possible signs of a stroke. It depends on which part of the brain is affected, and how severely, what signs or symptoms you will see. Many patients who have had a stroke present with chronic swelling of the foot, ankle, and leg on the affected side. This swelling is a hard, nonpitting type. It is caused because the muscles in the affected leg do not contract and work as they should. Muscle contracting helps to pump the tissue fluids back up the leg. Without this normal muscle contracture, the tissue fluids will pool in the foot and leg to cause the swelling.

A foot service can be of great benefit to the client who has had CVA. WARNING: Keep the foot soak water warm but not hot. Learn good massage techniques to help reduce the swelling and to improve the muscle tone. Recommend good skin care products. You will not cure this client but he or she will be extremely grateful for the care you give them.

L.O. 11

ARTERIOSCLEROSIS OBLITERANS ("HARDENING OF THE ARTERIES," ASO)

There are two main forms of arteriosclerosis:

——— L.O. 12

1. **Atherosclerosis**—formation of fatty plaques or deposits on the inner layer of the artery.

2. **Monckeberg's arteriosclerosis**—involves the calcification of the middle tissue layer of the artery.

Both of these processes cause thickening of the walls of the arteries resulting in the loss of elasticity and finally in the actual **occlusion** (blockage) of the artery. The process also weakens the wall of the artery. This weakened area of the wall may rupture or balloon out and form an **aneurysm**. Both forms of arteriosclerosis may be present in the same individual but in different arteries. The terms arteriosclerosis and atherosclerosis are often used interchangeably. For our discussion it does not matter which type is present. What does matter is that the condition results in the reduction of blood flow to the lower extremity and foot.

Development

The development of arteriosclerosis is associated with a number of risk factors: age and gender, **hypertension** (high blood pressure), cigarette smoking, diabetes mellitus, and family history (**genetics**). Of these, smoking, hypertension, and diabetes are the major risk factors. The disease is more predominant in men between the ages of 50 to 70. Women show an increased incidence after age 60 possibly related to the hormonal changes of menopause. High blood pressure increases the incidence of coronary artery disease. There has not been a proven direct relationship between hypertension and arteriosclerosis of the arteries in the lower extremities. Smoking has been proven to cause injury to the linings of the arteries, while also altering the function of the platelets. These conditions and lifestyles along with other changes within the blood enhance the probabilities of developing arteriosclerotic changes within the arteries. Diabetes, as we will discuss, makes any arteriosclerotic changes within the arteries become more severe and promotes the early development of this process. A family history of arteriosclerosis increases the probabilities of developing arteriosclerosis.

Know the risk factors for the development of arteriosclerosis.

——— L.O. 12

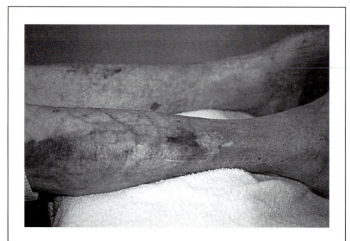

Figure 3-5 *Note the shiny and thin skin in the arteriosclerotic client. Underlying veins are easily observed. The slightest injury causes black and blue areas.*

Signs and Symptoms

The signs and symptoms of this disease are varied depending on its severity. For the purposes of this discussion we discuss those signs and symptoms that will indicate to the nail professional when *not* to perform a foot service.

Skin. The skin in advanced forms of arteriosclerosis becomes thin and shiny (Figure 3-5), as well as dry and cracked. The skin around the toes becomes tight and the fatty tissues within the toes and lower extremity begin to **atrophy**. The pulses in the foot may be absent. There is little or no hair growth on the foot or lower leg. The nails become brittle, thickened, and more susceptible to fungus infections. There may be open ulcers, usually over bony prominences or between the toes, which are extremely painful. These ulcers are particularly painful at night. This differentiates them from diabetic ulcers, which are pain free.

Pain. The presence of **ischemic** pain (pain caused by lack of oxygen to the tissues) is an indication of advanced arteriosclerosis. This pain is severe and unrelenting in nature. It may be much more severe at night because there is no muscle movement while sleeping to help force more blood through the hardened arteries to the tissues. This is typically called "rest pain." The client may explain the pain as being severe burning, tingling, stabbing, or a combination of these. Those clients with ischemic pain, particularly "rest pain," should not receive foot services from the nail professional. There is too great a risk of infections or the development of nonhealing wounds in these individuals.

Intermittent Claudication. Intermittent claudication may be a complaint of someone with arteriosclerosis. This condition is so named because it occurs intermittently with exercise and the word claudication in Latin means "to limp." The muscles of the legs cramp and ache while walking. These people must stop and rest the leg muscles before they can walk further. What they are experiencing is an ischemic type of pain in the muscles. Their arteries have become **sclerotic** (hardened) and cannot carry enough oxygenated blood to the tissues. The tissues become oxygen starved and cannot function normally. When the client stops exercising, in this case walking, the muscle tissues need less oxygen. In this nonexercising condition the diseased arteries are able to supply an adequate amount of oxygen to the muscles to reoxygenate them. After resting for a short time the individual may then continue walking until the muscles again begin to cramp and ache.

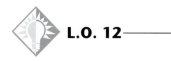

L.O. 12

Those clients with ischemic pain should not receive foot services from the nail professional.

These clients will tell you that they can walk only a specific distance, usually measured in city blocks or less, before they must stop and rest their legs. The distance they can walk is directly proportional to the severity of the disease process. The shorter the distance between rest stops the more severe the arteriosclerosis. Clients with complaints of inability to walk a block should be considered to have severe intermittent claudication and should not receive foot services in the salon setting.

Edema. Edema or swelling in the lower extremities may be a sign of advanced or severe arteriosclerosis. Some individuals, particularly the elderly, may sit for prolonged periods of time with their feet and legs in the **dependent position** (down). They may even sleep in a sitting position with their feet down. They do this unconsciously to get more blood to their legs and feet. Thus, there is less ischemic rest pain because fluid, in this case the needed blood, is helped into the area by force of gravity. The problem arises when the fluid portion of the blood (lymph) begins to pool in the lower extremity and is forced into the tissue spaces, resulting in edema.

The nail professional must be able to differentiate the edema of arteriosclerosis from that of other conditions, such as congestive heart failure, which cause swelling in the lower extremities, before making a decision about providing a foot service to a client with swelling in the feet and legs. This can be done by asking questions such as:

The nail professional must be able to differentiate the edema of arteriosclerosis from that of other conditions.

◆ When did the swelling start?

◆ Did it come on suddenly?

◆ Does the swelling go away after a night's sleep or is it still present in the morning on arising?

◆ Does the client have shortness of breath?

◆ Is any pain associated with the swelling?

Generally the swelling associated with conditions other than arteriosclerosis is painless, goes away after a night's sleep, and may come on fairly suddenly. The patient with congestive heart failure or emphysema will have shortness of breath and generalized fatigue. The opposite of these is generally true in the arteriosclerotic patients. Look for the skin changes seen with arteriosclerosis. Thin, shiny skin with atrophy or loss of fat in the underlying tissue is typical. The client with edema caused by arteriosclerosis should be referred out of the salon for foot care. The risks involved in providing the service outweigh benefits the nail professional may provide the client.

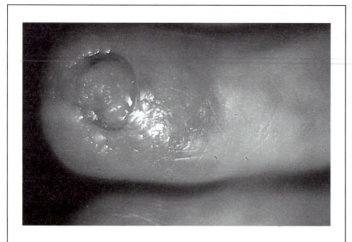

Figure 3-6 Blue toe. Notice a color change distal to where the small blood vessels have become blocked. The toe appears red but if the patient stands on the foot the color is bluish (cyanotic).

"Blue Toe" Syndrome. Another condition associated with arteriosclerosis, which may be observed in a salon setting, is the "blue toe" syndrome (Figure 3-6). There was once a patient who called a doctor's office complaining of a very painful ingrown toenail. She had been suffering with it for a number of weeks and that day decided she could no longer put up with the pain. They saw her that day in the office and examination found the entire big toe on her right foot to be cold and dark bluish in color. It actually looked about the color of a new pair of blue jeans. Her toenail was normal and not ingrown and no infection was present, but the toe was extremely painful. The rest of her foot was normal in color, warm, and pain free. Both pulses were present. She had no complaints of intermittent claudication. She did give a history of long-term one pack-a-day cigarette smoking. This patient had presented with the classic "blue toe" syndrome. They referred her to a vascular surgeon because the treatment involved is beyond the scope of podiatry care.

Blue toe does NOT refer to nail polish!

The "blue toe" syndrome is associated with atherosclerosis in the abdominal aorta or iliac arteries in the groin. Small **emboli** (blood clots, calcific plaques, or debris from the diseased wall of the artery) break away from the diseased area of the artery and become lodged in the small arterioles of the toes. In the above case it was the big toe but it can happen in any of the toes. The emboli cause a blockage in the arteriole, which results in an ischemic condition within the toe. The lack of blood and oxygen causes the toe to turn blue and become cold. If the process is not corrected gangrene (death of tissues) can be the end result. If you encounter this condition refer the client to a physician or podiatrist who will see that he or she receives proper care.

If the nail professional works closely with the arteriosclerotic clients, physician, or podiatrist, some foot services may be safely rendered in the salon setting. If you have any question about the client's condition check with the medical professionals before giving a service.

DIABETES MELLITUS

If any one systemic disease is the most important for the nail professional to be aware of, it is **diabetes**. Why? Diabetes causes any problem or disease process, no matter how small, to be exaggerated. An ingrown hair can become a massive infection. A small scrape or blister from an improperly fit shoe can lead to an amputation. Do we have your attention now? If so, let's discuss diabetes in general and identify those diabetics who may be safely serviced by the knowledgeable, well-trained nail professional.

One in 20 Americans has diabetes.

It is estimated that over 11 million individuals in the United States, or 1 in 20, have diabetes. There are many others who are diabetic who are not diagnosed. Once a man was brought into an office by his wife because she could no longer stand the odor emanating from his foot when he removed his shoe. She brought him into the office and on examination a large ulcer was found under the fifth metatarsal head of his right foot. The approximate diameter of this ulcer was the size of a dime and it had perforated through the skin into the underlying tissues (Figure 3-7). It was infected, had a foul odor, and was draining pus. The point of this is that he could not feel it! No one could walk on an ulcer such as this because it would be too painful. This patient had never been diagnosed as having diabetes nor had he had a physical examination by a physician in the last 5 years. With the presence of this pain-free ulcer, his doctor was certain that he was a diabetic. He was referred to his family physician for a work-up and subsequent laboratory tests confirmed his diabetic status. Once the diabetes was under control he was then able to control the infection and heal the ulcer, but it took well over a year.

It is estimated that 40% to 45% of the lower extremity amputations in the United States, which are not a result of injury, are the result of diabetic complications, primarily due to the diabetic's poor circulatory status and reduced ability to fight infections. Up to 20% of the burns treated on the feet are the result of the individual having diabetes and the resultant loss of feeling in the feet.
WARNING: Diabetic people are unable to feel that the water they are soaking their feet in is too hot or that they are being burned by the heating pad, which they are using to "warm" their feet. There have been third degree burns on the feet from soaking them in "hot water." Sleeping with the feet on a heating pad, even though it has been turned on a low setting, can

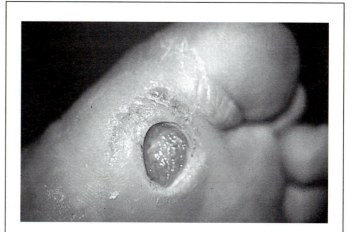

Figure 3-7 *Diabetic ulcer, approximately 2 cm in diameter. It penetrates through all layers of the skin into the subcutaneous tissues.*

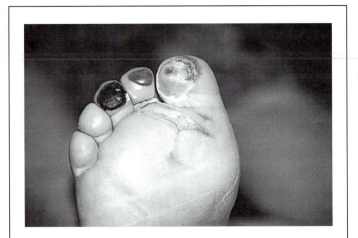

Figure 3-8 *Second and third degree burns on the bottom of a diabetic foot. The patient had cold feet and placed them over the floor heater. She then fell asleep with her feet on the heater and did not feel the burn happening.*

also cause severe burns on the insensitive foot (Figure 3-8).

Diabetes results from the body's inability to use blood sugar (glucose). This results from a decrease in the production of **insulin** by the **pancreas** or from the body developing a resistance to its own insulin. Insulin is a key ingredient that enables glucose to pass from the bloodstream into the surrounding tissue cells. A number of causes can decrease insulin production within the pancreas. The primary cause is genetic or an inherited trait that stops the production of insulin by the pancreas. Secondary causes include diseases of the pancreas such as infections. Injury to the pancreas from overuse of alcoholic beverages also results in a decrease of insulin production. Certain drugs, such as diuretics , cortisone, and thiazides (blood pressure medications), may also result in the decrease of insulin production. In rare instances, pregnancy may cause a glucose intolerance that results in a diabetic condition.

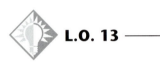 **L.O. 13**

Diabetes is subdivided into two categories. Type 1 is called insulin-dependent **diabetes mellitus** (IDDM) and type 2 is non-insulin-dependent diabetes mellitus (NIDDM). Type 1, at one time, was called juvenile diabetes but is now referred to as type I because it is not restricted to the juvenile age group. Approximately 30% of the diabetics in this category are diagnosed after the age of 30. Type 1 is characterized by sudden onset with symptoms being present for only a few days to a period of weeks. The classical symptoms are **polyuria** (excessive production of urine), **polydipsia** (excessive thirst), and **polyphagia** (excessive intake of food) are present in combination or singularly. Sudden weight loss is also typically found in these cases. **Ketoacidosis** (the excessive breakdown of protein or muscles within the body), which is potentially life threatening, may be in some cases the initial symptom. In the type 1 diabetic, the administration of insulin is necessary to maintain life and will be necessary for the rest of the individual's life.

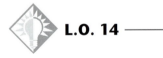 **L.O. 14**

Type 2 was formally referred to as adult-onset diabetes. It occurs in individuals over the age of 30, with the average age of diagnosis between 60 and 65 years. It is characterized by very gradual onset. It has been estimated that the disease process may be present for as long as 10 years before the diagnosis of diabetes is made in many of these individuals. This is like the man we discussed with the foot ulcer. The actual complications of diabetes may be the first symptoms of the disease. Type 2 diabetics actually produce insulin but for some reason their body develops a resistance to it. In some individuals, if the actual insulin levels are measured they may well be within normal limits. Diet, exercise, and oral diabetic medications can therefore control the blood sugar levels of type 2 diabetics. Some type 2 diabetics may become type 1 or insulin dependent as the disease progresses. Compared to type 1 diabetics, many individuals with type 2 disease can be classified as obese.

Diabetes is diagnosed by a laboratory test called the **oral glucose tolerance test**. This test consists of the administration of 75 grams of glucose, which is administered orally to the patient who has been fasting for the previous 12 hours. Before the test is administered, these patients have been advised to eat at least 150 to 200 grams of carbohydrates (sugars) daily for three days prior to the test. This is done to stress the individual's glucose-metabolizing system, thus giving a better test result. After the administration of the 75 grams of glucose, the blood sugar is measured at intervals over the next two hours. To make the diagnosis of diabetes, the blood sugar must be elevated above 200 at least once during the two-hour test and also at the end of the two hours. (Normal blood sugars run between 70 and 120 milligrams per deciliter [mg/dL] of blood.) The glucose tolerance test is administered to individuals who present with the classic symptoms of diabetes—the three "polys"—polyuria, polydipsia and polyphagia—and whose fasting blood sugar levels have been measured at greater than 140 mg/dL.

Once the diagnosis has been made, the patient will be classified type 1 or type 2. Depending on the classification, the blood sugars will be controlled through a combination of diet, exercise, and the use of oral medication or injectable insulin. Adequate control of the disease is obtained when the blood sugars are 150, or less, two hours after eating a meal. Blood sugar levels in poorly controlled diabetics can be as high as 300 to 400 mg/dL or over. In some uncontrolled diabetics, the blood sugar can actually go lower than normal (less than 70). The uncontrolled diabetic may exhibit symptoms that are termed diabetic shock and can actually lapse into a diabetic coma. This is a severe condition that must be treated immediately or it may result in death. Depending on whether the blood sugar is high or low, it either needs to be raised by the administration of glucose (oral or injected) or lowered by the administration of insulin. If you happen to be with an individual who is diabetic and he becomes confused, incoherent, and starts perspiring profusely, it is best to give him sugar in the form of orange juice or a candy bar and see that he obtains medical care. Even though he is diabetic, too much sugar will not cause as much harm as too little sugar as long as the individual receives medical care in a timely fashion. Most, but not all, diabetics will carry a candy bar or some other form of sugar with them and will recognize when their blood sugar is getting too low.

—— L.O. 15

Diet, exercise, and oral diabetic medications can therefore control the blood sugar levels of type 2 diabetics.

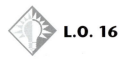

Diabetes affects the skin, vascular system, nerves, and pain sensation, especially in the feet.

Because of the abnormal **metabolism** of carbohydrates, fat, and protein, medically related problems are seen in the skin, and vascular and neurologic systems of the diabetic. These changes are accentuated by the disease process. The changes seen in these systems are generally more severely accentuated in the lower extremities.

The skin, because of the underlying vascular and neurologic changes, exhibits many diabetic-related changes. Dryness resulting in cracks, which may become infected, is one of the major changes. Generalized itching of the skin can also be a sign of diabetes. Because the skin is not healthy, it is more prone to fungal and yeast infections. Because of the lack of sensation, the skin is more prone to breakdown over pressure areas resulting in pain-free "diabetic ulcers." There is an increased incidence of the formation of corns and calluses because of the increased dryness of the skin. Toenails become thickened, yellow, and brittle and are also more prone to fungal and yeast infections.

The vascular system, for reasons not clearly understood, is severely affected by the disease. Arteriosclerotic changes in the arteries of the lower extremity are more common and more severe and occur earlier than in other areas of the body. The arterioles are first affected by the disease. Because the lower extremity has an abundant supply of arterioles, the early changes are seen in this area (Figure 3-9). Arteriosclerosis reduces the diameter of the arterioles or arteries, thus reducing the blood flow to the tissue. Because of the lack of proper nutrition to the tissues, the changes in the skin and neurologic systems are seen. The more the blood supply is reduced, the more prone the individual is to infections and gangrene, which ultimately results in an increased incidence of amputations in the diabetic population. Another reason, besides the decreased circulation, that the diabetic has a reduced ability to fight infections is because the disease reduces the effectiveness of white blood cells to fight infection. The white blood cell cannot readily engulf or **phagocytize** the bacteria or foreign substances, thus enabling the infection to spread and become more severe.

The nerves of the lower extremity become involved because of reduced blood supply and nutrition. Also, the sugar metabolism within the nerve is affected. This all results in a degeneration or injury of the nerve itself. Diabetic **neuropathy** ensues with all of the problems that go along with it. The neuropathy can be painful or painless. The actual loss of

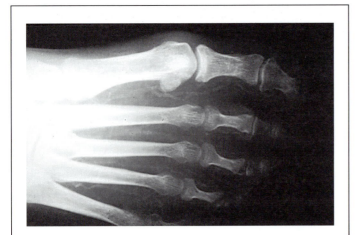

Figure 3-9 *X-ray of the foot of a 40-year-old diabetic. Notice the calcified arterioles between the metatarsals. They can even be observed extending into the toes! These calcified arterioles sometimes are seen in an 80-year-old's foot but almost never in someone age 40.*

feeling in the foot is most often an early finding of the disease itself. For the purposes of the nail professional, this is one of the most important findings you need to be aware of. Your service in the presence of this finding may be causing damage or injury without you or the client knowing it until it is too late. The sensation of pain is a protective mechanism. Pain tells us to pull our hand away from a hot pan or to stop doing whatever is causing the pain. In the absence of pain we continue doing those things, which in the end will cause a severe injury.

Remember the man with the foot odor who was walking on the infected ulcer that he did not feel? Another such incident was a diabetic patient who came in with what he thought to be an infected ingrown nail of his third toe. On examination, the nail appeared to be inflamed and had a slight drainage coming from under the nail plate. When trying to trim the nail, the nail nippers would not cut through it. On closer examination there was a broken piece of his insulin needle, about 3/8 inch long, that was jammed into his toe right under the toenail. Some way, he had driven this piece of needle under his toenail without even feeling it. The needle was easily removed and the infection healed with no serious consequences. This patient did not realize that he had lost feeling in his feet because the numbness had come on so gradually. He could not believe that he had a piece of his insulin needle under his toenail nor could he believe he could not even feel it! A client with a loss of feeling in the feet must be instructed to visually inspect the feet daily, looking for any cracks, open sores, or other injuries. This visual inspection will lead to an early detection of problems that might otherwise become more severe if left unattended (Figures 3-10 and 3-11).

Another severe problem in the **insensitive** foot is the so-called **Charcot joint**. This is a condition in which the bone around a weight-bearing joint becomes injured and actually begins to disintegrate. The patient does not feel the initial injury happening so he or she keeps walking on it and

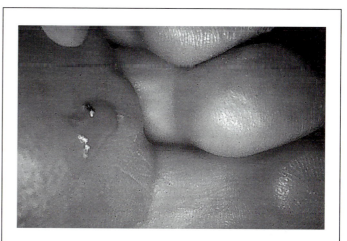

Figure 3-10 *This diabetic patient was having her routine foot care. A small black dot was seen on the ball of one foot. The area around it was slightly inflamed. When a small needle was used to probe the area, some pus and a wood sliver came out.*

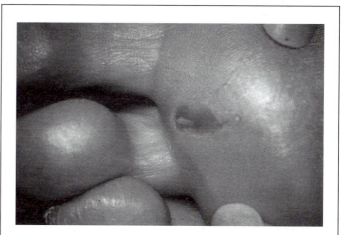

Figure 3-11 *After the overlying skin was debrided, a small ulcer was seen almost penetrating the entire depth of the skin. The patient had no idea there was an infection present much less that she had stepped on a wood sliver!*

the process becomes more severe to the point that the surrounding joints and bones also become affected, thus compounding this destructive process. The foot becomes extremely swollen and the skin temperature increases. This all happens without the patient ever feeling pain, other than an occasional ache or shooting pain that does not last. Without treatment, ulcers may develop and amputation will be the end result. Treatment consists of casting and keeping the patient non-weight-bearing until the bone repairs itself. Even after healing the foot will remain deformed and will not function properly.

Shoe fitting in the diabetic client is extremely important. Minor blisters or bruises from improperly fit shoes can become serious, devastating problems. A minor ingrown toenail without treatment can lead to an amputation. Conservative preventive care is the best safeguard against the devastating effects of diabetes. In no other disease is the old adage "prevention is worth a pound of cure" more true than in the diabetic. A team approach to the care of a diabetic is necessary. The medical doctor will control the disease itself. Specialists such as a podiatrist, dermatologist, vascular surgeon, and orthopedist will care for the more acute problems relating to their specialties that may arise. In selected cases, the nail professional can be an invaluable cost-effective member of this team in providing preventive foot care to the diabetic.

Now that we have talked about the serious consequences of diabetes let us discuss under what circumstances the well-trained, knowledgeable nail professional can safely provide services to the diabetic. Your initial history and personal evaluation are extremely important in making the determination as to whether to give or not to give a service to the diabetic client. After completing the history and personal evaluation on the type 1 or type 2 diabetic if you have any question at all about rendering the service *don't do it!* Contact that person's podiatrist and primary care doctor and discuss your concerns with them. Only after this discussion, and then only if they authorize the services you recommend, should you proceed with foot care for this client.

WARNING: When taking the client history and performing the personal evaluation on a diabetic you need to determine the following points. All of these must be evaluated before a decision can be made as to whether or not to provide a foot service to diabetic client.

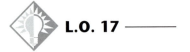 **L.O. 17**

◆ How is the diabetes controlled? Are they type 1 insulin dependent, or are they type 2 non-insulin dependent. If type 2 are they controlled by diet, exercise, oral medications, or a combination of the three? These questions will give you an idea of how severe the diabetes is. A type 2 diet and exercise-controlled diabetic may be treated like any other client. You should exercise more caution in performing your service and you must be on the look out for any small problems that you might well overlook in your nondiabetic clients.

- The type 1 insulin-controlled diabetics, as well as type 2 diabetics taking oral medication to control blood sugar, must be further evaluated before a foot service is given.

- How long have they been diabetic? The longer an individual is a diabetic the more progressive are the changes seen in the skin, nerves, and blood vessels.

- How often do they check the urine or blood for sugar? This question will help you to determine if they are serious about the disease by keeping regular track of how well under control the diabetes is. If they never or infrequently test themselves you need to determine why. Has their doctor told them that it is not necessary for them to do it? Do they not check it because they forget or are they in denial about their disease? If their doctor told them not to test that is one thing. If they are ambivalent about their disease, you do not want to take any responsibility for these clients. Refer them to their podiatrist or primary physician for foot care.

- What is their usual blood sugar level when they test it? Knowing what their average blood sugar is will be a big factor in helping you to determine whether or not to provide services to these clients. Remember the normal blood sugar levels are between 70 and 120 mg/dL. To be under adequate control a diabetic's blood sugar should be stable and run between 150 to 200 mg/dL. Therefore, if your clients have sugar levels over 200 mg/dL you should not assume any responsibility for their foot care. They should be referred to their podiatrist.

The longer an individual is a diabetic the more progressive are the changes.

- When performing the personal evaluation, check the condition of the skin. Is it dry with open cracks? Are there any blisters, open wounds, ulcers, or infections (bacterial or fungus)? Is the skin red and shiny, which can indicate poor circulation? What is the skin temperature—cold or warm? Cold may indicate reduced circulation. Are there areas of pressure callus formation on the toes, heels, or the balls of the feet? If so these are prone to pressure sores and ulcers. Do not forget to check between the toes for cracks, soft corns, fungus infections or other potentially serious problems. Note these on your form for future reference. If any of these skin conditions are present a podiatric or dermatologic referral is necessary. Depending on the severity of these conditions you may be able to work with the client's doctors in maintaining foot health by routine pedicures once the acute problems are handled.

◆ Check the circulatory status. Can you feel the two pulses in each foot? Check the **capillary filling time** by compressing the skin over the big toe and then releasing the pressure. The underlying tissues that were compressed will be white or blanched out because the blood was squeezed out of the capillaries. The time it takes for the blood to return to the area, which is indicated by the tissues becoming pink again, is called the capillary filling time. It should take less than 30 seconds for the tissues to become pink again. If it takes longer do not give a pedicure service.

◆ What color are the underlying tissues if the feet are in the dependent position? Purplish blue (cyanotic) or deep reddish (rubor) in color? Both of these indicate lack of oxygen to the tissues, most probably because of arteriosclerotic changes in the arteries, and are symptoms of an impaired circulatory status. Ask clients if they experience any muscle fatigue or cramping when they are walking or climbing stairs. If they answer yes, and tell you they can only walk a block and then have to stop and rest because the muscles in their legs ache, they have intermittent claudication, which may indicate advanced arteriosclerotic changes in the vessels. In the presence of any of the above negative findings you should not give a foot service to the diabetic client.

◆ Check the neurologic status. The main thing here is to determine whether clients have lost any of the feeling in their feet. Do this by lightly rubbing the bottom of the foot with your hand. Then with the same pressure rub the client's arm or leg. If they report that they feel it more in the arm or leg than the foot they probably are experiencing some form of diabetic neuropathy. This is a very rough test; however, it can give an idea about whether the client has lost any of the feeling in the foot. Individuals who have a loss of feeling in their feet should not receive a foot service from the nail professional. It is too easy to cause an injury, no matter how slight, to the insensitive foot. The liability involved is not worth the risk. Refer such clients to the podiatrist for their foot care.

By understanding the basics of diabetes you will be better able to assess your clients' needs for foot services and products. You will be able to discuss your clients' problems, in a knowledgeable manner, with their medical professionals should the occasion require. You will be better equipped to be a member of the team of professionals giving care, in individual areas of specialization, to the needs of diabetic clients.

The main thing is to determine whether clients have lost any of the feeling in their feet.

FOOT NOTES

Systemic diseases are those diseases that affect the entire body. Anyone who gives foot care or services must be aware of how these diseases affect the foot. Signs and symptoms of these diseases can be observed in the feet and legs. Be aware of them!

Of all of the systemic diseases diabetes causes more nontraumatic amputations than any other. Besides the loss of feeling, other problems such as arteriosclerosis, infections, and skin problems all can have devastating effects for the diabetic. The nail professional must be ever vigilant for the signs of diabetes when giving nail services to clients. The importance of taking and recording a thorough client history and personal evaluation cannot be overstressed. Remember average type 2 diabetic patients are not diagnosed until after they have had the disease for 10 years! Considering this and the fact that 1 in every 20 people within our society is diabetic, how many clients do you have who may fit into this statistic? If you follow the outline in this chapter, be aware of signs and symptoms, and never give a service if you have a question about the status of a client, you can safely give services to selected diabetic clients.

QUESTIONS

1. What is a systemic disease?

2. What is scleroderma?

3. What are the two types of arthritis and how do they affect the bone?

4. Rheumatoid arthritis is what type of arthritis? Osteoarthritis is
   what type?

5. What is ischemic pain?

6. If you see 40 clients how many of those *may* be diabetic?

7. What medication is used to control type 1 diabetes?

8. How are the arteries affected by diabetes? Which arteries are
   affected first?

9. Why is it important for diabetics to visually inspect their feet
   every day?

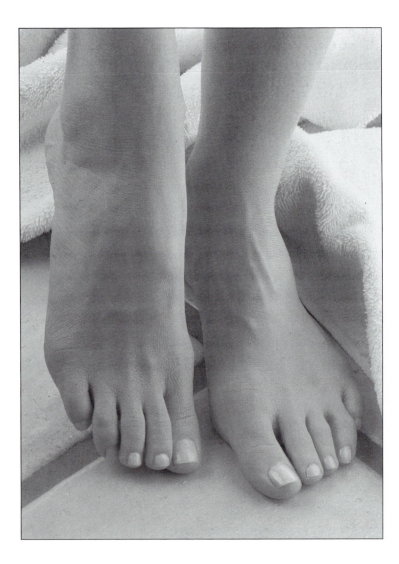

Common Foot Problems | 4

LEARNING OBJECTIVES

After studying this chapter, the reader should be able to:

1. Define and describe the gait cycle.

2. Describe an abnormally pronated foot and its treatment.

3. Briefly discuss the history of footwear, particularly three American innovations.

4. Differentiate between the two basic devices for measuring feet.

5. Relate the "Golden Rule" of skin disorders.

6. Describe friction blisters and their treatment.

7. Describe calluses and their treatments.

8. Differentiate between hard and soft corns and describe their treatment.

9. Describe warts, their cause and treatment.

10. Discuss how fungal infections are acquired.

11. Describe tinea pedis infections and their treatment.

12. Describe bacterial infections of the foot and differentiate these from fungal infections.

13. Compare and contrast hyperhidrosis, bromhidrosis, and anhidrosis.

14. Distinguish between primary and secondary contact dermatitis.

15. Describe chilblain and frostbite and their treatments.

16. Differentiate a pigmented nevus from a malignant melanoma and describe their treatments.

17. Describe the process that creates psoriasis.

18. *Describe two arch deformities and their treatments.*

19. *Distinguish hammertoe, mallet toe, congenital overlapping fifth toe, and hallux valgus with bunion and describe their treatments.*

20. *Discuss the causes of cold feet or burning feet.*

21. *Describe neurofibromas, their cause, symptoms, and treatment.*

22. *Discuss the usual cause of heel pain.*

This chapter should be used as a reference for localized conditions that you will encounter on the foot itself. It is essential to remember that most of the problems that occur locally on or in the foot are the result of the mechanical forces that the foot must withstand during walking. A good understanding of how the foot helps to propel us from one step to the next, known as the **"gait cycle,"** is necessary to understand why these conditions occur in the foot. If you understand this concept most of the misinformation and mystery about the causes of foot problems such as corns, calluses, hammertoes, and bunions will be answered for you. The history of footwear, proper shoe fitting, and the relationship of shoes to foot problems are also discussed.

THE GAIT CYCLE

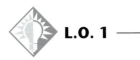 L.O. 1 ——————

We touched on the gait cycle at the beginning of Chapter 2. We will now discuss it more fully to better understand the foot and its function during walking. The foot is a dynamic organ. By this we mean that it serves more than one function and must make a smooth transition between functions while it is preforming its job. Without changing in a precise manner from one function to another, many uncomfortable circumstances will result.

The two basic functions of the foot during walking are adapting to the surface that is being walked on and propelling the body forward for the next step. Thus the two phases of the gait cycle (Figure 4-1) are termed the *adaptive phase* and the *propulsive phase*. In the adaptive phase the foot contours to the weight-bearing surface to prevent injury to itself. During the propulsive phase it becomes a rigid lever that allows it to push the body forward. This is a very basic explanation of the gait cycle, but for purposes of this book it is enough to assist you in understanding the basic cause of many abnormal foot conditions.

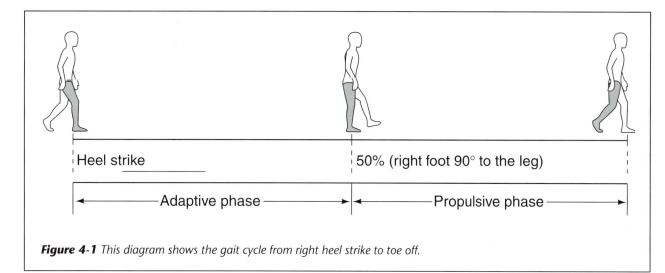

Heel strike

50% (right foot 90° to the leg)

←———Adaptive phase———→ ←———Propulsive phase———→

Figure 4-1 *This diagram shows the gait cycle from right heel strike to toe off.*

Adaptive Phase

The adaptive phase of the cycle begins when the heel makes contact with the surface being walked on. It ends when the leg is at a 90° angle to the foot. It allows the foot to adapt to the surface on which it will be resting. If one were walking on a rocky beach and the foot were rigid, it would become a very painful process. Extreme care would be needed not to step in such a manner as to injure the foot. To make walking easier and more efficient nature has developed a mechanism that allows the foot to become a loose bag of bones. This allows it to contour to the weight-bearing surface as we step on it.

To allow this to happen there must be a locking and unlocking mechanism within the foot. The unlocking mechanism is called **pronation**, which is a complex motion that occurs in the subtalar joint or the joint between the talus and the calcaneous. The actual motions in the foot that comprise pronation are **eversion**, **abduction**, and **dorsiflexion**. The amount of pronation necessary to unlock the foot is small, approximately 4°. It is when pronation extends beyond 4° that problems begin to arise in the foot.

You can compare the act of pronation in a foot to the shock absorbers and springs in a car. The shocks and springs allow the car to accommodate or adapt to any irregularities in the road. They give us a smooth ride over bumps and potholes so that we are not jarred around or injured while riding in the car. When our foot pronates it basically does the same job by allowing the foot to accommodate or adapt to any irregularities in the surface on which we are walking. The act of pronation in the foot reduces the potential for injury during the initial or adaptive phase of gait.

In pronation, our feet act like the shock absorbers and springs in a car—they adapt to any irregularities!

Propulsive Phase

During the last part of the adaptive phase the foot should have begun **inversion**, **adduction**, and **plantarflexion** motions that are the exact opposite of the motions of pronation. These motions when looked at as one are called **supination**, which is the locking motion. Try to remember this word by thinking of drinking soup out of your hand. If you make a spoon out of your hand you must move it into a supinated position. The motion in the foot is basically the same; however, it would be quite difficult to drink soup with your foot!

When the leg becomes perpendicular, or 90° to the foot, the foot should no longer be pronated or unlocked. It should be in a neutral or "locked" position. At this point all of the joints of the foot should align and lock to make the foot into a rigid lever. This rigid lever can then propel the body forward for the next step. This then starts the propulsive phase of gait. It is at this point many foot abnormalities begin to arise. If all 33 joints are not functioning as one rigid structure or lever during this phase of gait, the force of body weight begins to cause damage within the various structures of the foot.

Under usual circumstances the force exerted on the bottom of the foot during normal walking is approximately 25,000 pounds per square inch (psi). Any added strain exerted because of the lack of proper function adds many thousands of pounds to this figure. This extra force magnifies small problems that then manifest themselves over a period of time into the abnormal conditions that we see. Calluses, hammertoes, bunions, neuromas, ingrown nails, and many other foot abnormalities to be discussed arise because the foot remains abnormally pronated during the propulsive phase of gait. The foot instead of being a rigid lever arm remains a loose bag of bones, which over a period of time breaks down.

Flat Foot? Pronated Foot?

What the untrained individual generally calls a "flat foot" is usually an abnormally pronated foot. The pronated foot in the weight-bearing position appears to have no medial longitudinal arch, thus the misconception that this is a flat foot. If a pronated foot is observed in a non-weight-bearing circumstance an arch is easily identifiable. A true flat foot (congenital flat foot, or one with which the person is born) in a non-weight-bearing condition has no easily identifiable longitudinal arch. A true flat foot in most instances has fewer mechanically induced problems than the abnormally pronated foot. This is because the bony structures were already adapted at birth to a nonarched structure rather than the so-called normal foot that has an arch.

Another easy way to identify an abnormally pronated foot is to observe a standing individual from the back. The bottom of the heel will be pointed away from the midline of the body (this is an everted position in relation to the midline). Also the inside of the foot will appear to be protruding

The foot is receiving 25,000 pounds per square inch during normal walking!

L.O. 2 ————

medially (toward the midline of the body) and there will be minimal to no longitudinal arch present (Figure 4-2).

We have talked mainly about how the abnormally pronated foot is responsible for many foot problems. If we consider that the foot is really the foundation on which the rest of the body is supported we must also discuss the problems above the foot associated with this support. Our discussion of the pronated foot would not be complete unless we discussed problems of the body as a whole that are associated with abnormal foot function.

One of the first signs of a bad foundation under a house is that the roof sags. This is

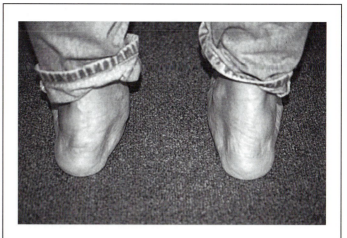

Figure 4-2 *The left foot is pronated while the right is in a normal weight-bearing position. The heel on the left is everted while that on the right is vertical.*

also true with the pronated foot. Many cases of chronic low back pain and fatigue can be directly associated with the pronated foot. Individuals such as cosmetologists and barbers who work standing may complain of these symptoms if their feet are abnormally pronated. They may find themselves at times unconsciously standing on the outside of their feet. What they are doing is supinating (the opposite of pronation) their feet, which causes an external rotation of the leg, which, in turn, causes a relaxation of some of the muscles in the low back. This in turn helps to relieve low back fatigue and pain. Some **sciatic nerve** pain in the legs may be caused or aggravated by abnormally pronated feet.

Treatment of the Abnormally Pronated Foot

Proper foot function is extremely important to the health of the foot as well as to the health of the body to which it is attached. Some patients will complain, when doing the initial history and physical, that they only came in for care of a foot problem. They may feel that you do not need to know about the rest of their medical conditions. Patiently explain to them that as long as their feet are connected to their body it is necessary to know all about them to treat their feet properly. Then educate them about problems such as we have discussed. Explain how these problems may relate to their feet. Never forget as you give a foot service that the foot is attached to an individual. Most individuals have no idea about how the feet function in relation to the rest of the body.

The treatment of the pronated foot is directed toward making it function within a normal range of motion, that is, it should be approximately 4° pronated at heel strike. It should then supinate and return to the "locked" or neutral position by the time the leg is at a 90° angle to the foot. In the abnor-

——— **L.O. 2**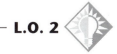

mally pronated foot this can be accomplished in a number of ways. The most accepted method is through the use of an **orthotic** device that is inserted into the shoe.

A short discussion is necessary here to clarify the difference between an arch support and an orthotic. An arch support is an over-the-counter product and it is generally premolded and fit to the shoe instead of to the foot. A variation of this occurs when the client steps onto an impression material (paper or foam) and from this a premolded arch support is fitted and dispensed. A true orthotic is a *custom prescription device* constructed to a corrected cast of the patient's foot. This cast is taken with the foot in the neutral position. The orthotic constructed on the neutral position cast allows for the normal motions to take place within the foot and stops the abnormal motions.

An arch support will in some cases work as well as an orthotic. When it does work it is usually in those individuals who do not have a severely pronated foot. An arch support may be tried as an initial treatment for certain foot conditions such as mild generalized foot pain. If the arch support does not help or helps only a small amount then an orthotic is the treatment of choice. Many arch supports are advertised and sold as orthotics. These devices are being sold over-the-counter at beauty shows and fairs. Remember the difference between an arch support and the orthotic and you will not be fooled by these inaccurate advertising claims.

It can be stated without reservation that the podiatrist is the best trained professional in the understanding of normal and abnormal foot biomechanics. The neutral position cast is absolutely necessary to the construction of a properly functioning orthotic. It takes someone who can scientifically determine the neutral position of the different foot types to properly perform this casting technique and the podiatrist is second to none in this process. If any of your clients have conditions similar to those we are discussing your referral to a podiatrist will be of benefit to them! They will appreciate the fact that you are a knowledgeable professional who understands and cares about their problems.

As we continue this chapter we will identify foot conditions that are caused or aggravated by the abnormally pronated foot.

A true orthotic is a custom prescription device constructed to a corrected cast of the patient's foot.

FOOT NOTES

The foot must function in a very precise manner. If it does not many abnormal problems result. The gait cycle is divided into two distinct phases—the adaptive phase and the propulsive phase. During the adaptive phase the foot accommodates to the surface being walked on. This minimizes the potential for injury to the foot. To allow accommodation the foot pronates to unlock the joints so that it is not a rigid and unyielding structure. It becomes a "loose bag of bones." The total amount of pronation needed to unlock the foot is only 4°. The propulsive phase starts when the leg is 90° to the foot. At this point the foot must be rigid to propel the body forward for the next step. The locking motion of the foot is called supination. When the foot remains pronated during the propulsive phase many common foot problems such as corns, callouses, neuromas, bunions, hammertoes, and ingrown nails result.

The treatment of the abnormally pronated foot is best accomplished with a prescription orthotic made from a neutral position cast of the foot. This prescription device allows the normal motions of pronation and supination to occur during the gait cycle.

SHOES

Did you know that for every one inch of heel height approximately 25% more pressure is transferred to the ball of the foot? This means if you wear a two-inch heel the ball of your foot is carrying 50% more pressure than it would if you were wearing flat shoes!

The pounds per square inch carried on the bottom of the foot is 25,000! Thus, a two-inch heel will add 12,500 psi to the pressure on the ball of the foot for a phenomenal 37,500 psi. No wonder women as a group have more foot complaints than men when one considers that approximately 59% of women wear high heels every day. The extra stress caused by this style of shoe contributes to, but is not the sole cause of, the development of bunions, hammertoes, neuromas, and other foot abnormalities.

For every one inch of heel height approximately 25% more pressure is transferred to the ball of the foot.

History

The first shoes were probably worn by our ancestors who lived in colder climates more than 12,000 years ago. These first shoes were probably a moccasin type made of leather, lined with fur or grass for insulation, wrapped around the foot, and held in place with a leather thong. They were to protect

——— **L.O. 3**

the foot from the cold rather than from the rocky harsh terrain they were walking on.

Sandals appear to be the next development in foot coverings. Pictures dating back 6000 to 9000 years BC show craftsmen constructing this type of "shoe." The earliest existent example of this is an Egyptian sandal dating back 2000 years BC. The sole was made of woven papyrus grass and it is utilitarian in nature. From this simple design the Egyptians and Mesopotamians introduced fashion by adding color, ornamentation, and different shapes to their sandals. From these simple beginnings arose shoe fashion as we know it today.

All footwear fashion comes from only seven basic designs: the moccasin, sandal, boot, pump, oxford, mule, and clog. The laced oxford is the newest of these and dates back 300 years! Also not one of these seven basic designs were created by or for women even though variations of these fashions for women have far outnumbered those for men. The 16th century introduced the "high heel" shoe into women's fashion, when Catherine de Medici, an Italian of 17, was sent to marry King Henry II of France. Because of her short stature she wore shoes designed with heels that added two to three inches to her height. They became a sensation of the time because of how they made her hips produce a seductive sway when she walked or danced. High heels became the rage of Europe to the point that the church clergy branded them "devices of Satan to stir the lusts of men." As late as 1770, New Jersey adopted an English law that stated that: "Any woman who, through the use of high-heeled shoes or other such devices, leads a subject of her majesty into marriage, shall be punished with the penalties of witchery." Massachusetts also had a similar law. How times change!

All shoes come from seven basic designs— from moccasins to clogs.

Early 19th century America gave the world three great innovations in the construction and fit of foot wear. Prior to then all shoes were made in "straight" **lasts** (the mold over which shoes are constructed). This allowed the shoe to be worn on either foot. This made shoes extremely hard to break in and many foot problems were directly attributable to the "straight" last shoe. The idea of a left and right shoe was first introduced in 1824 but was rejected by the public because the shoes looked "crooked." The Civil War saw a resurgence of the left and right shoe because soldiers of the Union Army demanded more comfortable shoes in which to march. After the war, shoe manufacturers returned to the "straight" last for economic reasons. It required only half as many lasts to produce shoes! It was not until about 1900 that the left and right shoe style reappeared on a full scale basis in the commercial marketplace.

The second thing that revolutionized shoe manufacturing was Elias Howe's invention of the sewing machine in 1846. This allowed the upper

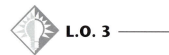 **L.O. 3**

pieces of the shoe to be sewn by machine instead of by hand. McKay then invented the sewing machine to stitch the sole to the upper part of the shoe. For the first time in history the mass production of footwear made shoes affordable to the general population.

The third innovation was the first rational system of shoe sizing put forth by Edwin B. Simpson of New York in 1886. Until this time shoes were generally available in only two sizes, large and small, fat or slim, or men's and women's. Simpson's system of progressive measurements applied separately to men's, women's, children's, and infant's lasts. He based his system on one-third of an inch for each full size change in length. In other words, if you change from a size 6 to a size 7 the actual addition in length is one-third of an inch. To change a half size (6 to 6 1/2) the actual length of change is only one-sixth of an inch!

Under Simpson's system the ball width measurement is one-fourth of an inch to the size. In other words, a change from width A to B equals one-fourth of an inch. An AA width, therefore, would be approximately one-eighth of an inch narrower than an A width. This system finally gave the world uniformity in shoe sizing and by the turn of the century it was in full use. In theory this is great! However, read on.

The bad news! Today we seem to be going back to the 18th century as far as fitting shoes is concerned. Stores, because of economics, are only stocking certain sizes and widths. Because of these demands manufacturers are only manufacturing those sizes and widths that the shoe stores are requesting. Half sizes are becoming a thing of the past. Instead of 14 widths (AAAAA to EEEEE) we now have N (narrow), M (medium), and W (wide). There are few if any combination lasts, that is, A width at the ball and AA width at the heel. Under the Simpson system of shoe sizing there are theoretically 300 different sizes available. Today in 95% of the shoe stores, only a small fraction of these combinations is available for the consumer. To add to the problem, some stores carry only one or two widths (N and W, or only M). They also carry only those lengths that are the most common (6 to 9 for women, and 9 to 12 for men).

Another complicating factor in fitting shoes is the last. The last actually determines the shape and internal volume of the shoe. Each different shoe manufacturer has its own different lasts for its different styles of shoes. A size 6B in one manufacturer's shoe may be a 7A in another manufacturer's shoe. It should tell you to never go by size when fitting different brands of shoes. The actual measurement of your foot is only a starting point in obtaining a properly fit shoe. This gives added meanings to the old adage "If the shoe fits, wear it."

The actual difference between shoe sizes may be small, but it can make a BIG difference in fit and comfort!

Shoe Fitting

In reality fitting shoes is not that much of a mystery. The basic thing is to use your head and not your emotions when buying shoes. Look at the shoe and then look at your foot. Do they even remotely match? If not check out another shoe of a different style or type. Do not squeeze your foot into something in which it does not belong. You are only asking for trouble later! Another thing to remember is that there are well over 230,000 shoe salesmen or women out there just waiting for you to enter their stores. Fewer than 10% of these salespeople have ever had any training in basic foot anatomy or in how to size or fit the shoe. Many, if not the majority, are paid by commission. This means that unless they sell you a pair of shoes they do not get paid or at least they do not make as much money. This gives an incentive to sell the shoes whether they fit or not. How many times have you been told, "The shoe will stretch after you have worn it for a while." If you hear that statement, run, don't walk, out of the store because that salesperson is trying to sell a shoe for the commission and not for your comfort. Never purchase a pair of shoes with the hopes that they will feel better after you have worn them for a while. They should fit comfortably when you leave the store. Make it a habit to shop only in stores that offer at least three widths, preferably more, in most all of the styles that they offer.

Match your foot and desired shoe — but use your head!

L.O. 4 —————— Always remember, never tell salespersons your size! They are there to fit you properly and part of that fitting requires them to measure your feet (yes, this means both feet) for size. There are two basic measuring devices used in most shoe stores. One is a ruler or size-stick device that basically measures the length of the foot from the back of the heel to the end of the toes. The other is the Brannock device, which more accurately measures the size of the foot (Figure 4-3). The Brannock device measures the length of the foot from heel to ball, as well as from heel to toe. It also measures the width of the foot at the same time. Put more faith in the stores using the Brannock device because it shows that they care more about getting a proper fit for their customers. Either of these measuring devices only gives us a starting point from which to get a proper fit. Remember the difference in the lasts!

Once your foot has been measured then you can start trying shoes. Remember we have first looked at the shoe and compared it to our foot. We have then had our foot measured for length, heel to ball and heel to toe, as well as

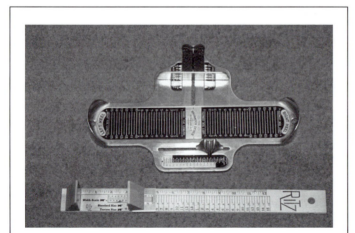

Figure 4-3 *The Brannock (upper) and the size-stick (lower) foot measuring devices*

width. We are now going to try on the shoe. The first thing to check is the heel to ball length. Do this by standing up (this puts weight on the foot and lengthens it), leaning over and placing your thumb at that point of the shoe where if you moved your thumb back toward the arch the shoe would get narrower and if you moved your thumb forward toward the end of your toes the shoe would also become narrower. This is the widest part of the shoe and your thumb nail should be centered on it (Figure 4-4). You should be able to feel your first metatarsal head (the bump of bone on the side of your foot that your big toe connects to), centered under your thumb. If you do, you now have the widest part of the shoe corresponding to the widest part of your foot.

Next, check where the ends of your toes are in relationship to the end of the shoe. If the shoe is the proper length your toes will be nowhere near the end of the shoe. The exception to this is if you have long slender toes. In this case you may have to fit your shoes heel to toe rather than heel to ball. In any case try to leave half an inch or about a thumb width between the end of the toe and the end of the shoe.

The big trick is to now get the proper width so that you will not slip back and forth in the shoe. This is accomplished by trial and error. If your foot has been measured a C start at that width and walk around the store in the shoes. If they slip in the heel they are too wide and you must try narrower sizes. If they pinch in the ball of the foot it is too narrow so you must try a wider width. When you have followed these instructions and if the shoe feels good on your foot you have found the "proper fit" for that particular style and last. If the shoe fits and you are happy with it, buy it! It will be comfortable and most likely will not cause any added foot problems.

Know how to properly fit shoes, for yourself and to educate your clients.

What to Wear—Style Versus Comfort

High-heeled fashion pump style shoes are made to look at and not to wear!! They are not even remotely shaped like the human foot and in wearing them you might as well be standing on the side of a mountain with your toes pointed downhill all day long—notwithstanding the fact that for every one inch of heel height added you add an extra 25% more pounds per square inch to the 25,000 psi the ball of the foot already normally carries. Also the only way these shoes will stay on the foot is by squeezing the ball and toes of the foot and by pinching the heel. Basically the shoe holds onto the foot like a

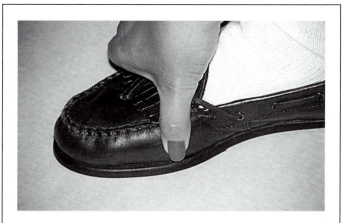

Figure 4-4 *The thumb nail is centered over the head of the first metatarsal and at the widest point of the shoe. From this point the shoe gets narrower toward the toes and from here it also gets narrower toward the heel.*

vice. It must be said here that flats or stylish pump-like shoes without heels are the same. The only thing they do differently from heels is that they do not add the extra pressure to the ball of the foot.

> *Look for the shoe to have as much padding and support as possible in the ball of the shoe as well as in the arch.*

For some reason women think small feet look more feminine. This style of shoe makes feet look smaller by placing the foot in a more vertical position and by constricting the foot three-quarters to an inch in width to make it look narrower. These shoes will ultimately aggravate or cause pain under the metatarsal heads (metatarsalgia). Bunions, hammertoes, calluses, ingrown nails, thick toe nails, corns, neuromas, blisters, and many other problems are caused by this style of shoe. These conditions, if present at all, in all probability would not bother the wearer if they were in a shoe style that was made to fit the human foot. Realize women are going to wear this style of shoes and let's see if we can get some semblance of fit or comfort with them.

The pump style "heel," or pump style "flat" cannot be fit in the same manner already discussed. Remember they have to fit like a vice to stay on the foot, so let's try to get as comfortable a vice as possible. The "pointed toe" style may look fashionable but is your foot pointed? For working shoes, in these styles, try to get a rounded, squared-off toe box style. For a working shoe do not select one where the upper part of the shoe is sewn into the sole so that it is a wedge shape for the toes to fit into. Save the pointed toe styles for parties or special events where you do not have to wear them too long. Also for working shoes, in these styles, try not to get over 1 to 1 1/2 inch heel. Better yet, get a pump style flat! Look for the shoe to have as much padding and support as possible in the ball of the shoe as well as in the arch. Try to purchase shoes with soles of crepe rubber, rubber, or a material of sufficient thickness to give good shock absorption and protection to the ball of the foot during walking or standing.

Some companies manufacture athletically designed high-heeled shoes or walking pumps. These are similar to the classic high heel but offer more cushioning, shock absorption, and support. Comparison studies have shown them to offer more comfort than their classic counterparts. None of these are recommended as a "walking" shoe. Walking shoes are flat and should be fit as first described. The athletic shoe companies all have "walking" shoes and they are recommended highly for this purpose. If you work in a job where you stand for long periods of time, do not wear heels. If you can, wear a nurse style or athletic style walking shoe. If you cannot wear either of these then at least wear an athletically designed pump style flat.

—— *If the Shoe Fits,* Godfrey F. Mix, D.P.M. (*NAILS*, Bobit Publishing, Redondo Beach, CA, Dec. 1994, pages 40-46). Reprinted with permission of the publisher. Copyright © 1994 *NAILS Magazine.*

FOOT NOTES

Use your head not your emotions when purchasing shoes! Shop only in shoe stores that offer at least three widths in the styles of shoes that they stock. Do not tell the salesperson your size. He or she should measure both of your feet, and if not, find another store. Remember the measurement is only a starting point. Different lasts and brands will fit differently for each person. Fit shoes first from heel to ball unless you have long slender toes—then you must fit heel to toe. Next fit for width so the shoes do not slip around.

Be aware that pump style heels or flats do not fit the human foot. They are "devices of Satan." Fit them so they do not fall off and use the guidelines we have outlined when purchasing them. Wear them as little as possible remembering that they cause or aggravate many painful foot conditions. Just because a shoe costs a lot of money does not mean it is a better shoe for your foot or that it will fit you better. You are basically paying for better materials that should wear longer. You may also be paying for a brand name or a particular style. As a general statement wear the shoe that is designed for the type of activity you are participating in. In the end the shoe is only a protective covering for the foot. Be sure it fits no matter what you wear!

Dr. William Scholl made the following slogan a household expression: "When your feet hurt, you hurt all over!" Think about this when purchasing your shoes and follow the old adage "If the shoe fits wear it." You will live a more pleasant, healthy, and comfortable life in a shoe that fits your foot!

As a beauty professional who gives foot services discuss proper footwear with your clients. Demonstrate to them that you are knowledgeable in the area of shoes and shoe fitting. Talk to those around you in the beauty salon about foot comfort and shoes. Make recommendations to them on shoe types and fitting. Be a teacher and you will receive back much more than you give. Last but not least, have fun shoe shopping!

Just because a shoe costs a lot of money does not mean it is a better shoe for your foot or that it will fit you better.

CONDITIONS OF THE SKIN

The skin as the outer covering of the foot is subject to many different kinds of injuries and stresses than the skin of other parts of our body. Some of the common skin problems and a few of the not so common problems are discussed in this section.

You may want to review the section on the skin in Chapter 2. The skin on the soles of the feet is extremely thick in comparison to other areas. There are many sweat glands located on the bottom of the foot. Disorders such as **bromidrosis** (smelly feet) may result. There are few sebaceous glands in the skin of the foot so the skin here will have more of a tendency to dry and crack. Internal fluid pressure is extreme in the foot because it is the lowest part of the body. This causes extra stress on the skin resulting in conditions such as stasis dermatitis or stasis ulcers.

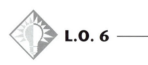

L.O. 5

Never forget the "Golden Rule" for providing service to clients with skin disorders.

The "Golden Rule" of skin disorders states "if the area of skin to be worked on is infected, inflamed, broken, or raised (swollen) a nail technician should not service the client."[1] This is a good rule to observe in giving a foot service. In my opinion however, some foot services may be rendered in the presence of swelling. If the nail professional is aware of the cause of the swelling, a foot service may be rendered if it will not cause harm to the client. We have already discussed this in conditions such as congestive heart failure and swelling caused by arteriosclerosis. The services must be tailored to the individual and as emphasized must cause no harm or aggravate the condition causing the swelling. Of course if the swelling is from an injury, an infection, or from an unknown cause the "Golden Rule" must apply.

Friction Blister

L.O. 6

Friction blisters are just what the name implies. They are a localized reaction of the skin to friction from an external source. They are the most common reaction of the skin to trauma. They are really only seen in the human species. In the foot they are most commonly caused by the rubbing of shoes. Improper mechanics of the foot during walking can also be a cause. In this case the sole of the foot is most usually involved.

Friction blisters are filled with a straw-colored tissue fluid. This fluid collects in the space created by the injury to the skin just below the stratum granulosum or middle layer of the skin. It is best not to break the blister but rather to let it heal within itself. If the blister does break before it is healed then a topical antibiotic ointment and a dressing should be applied until it

---

[1]Milady's Art and Science of Nail Technology, Albany, NY: Milady Publishing rev. ed., 1997, pp 65 and 78.

is healed. An open blister particularly on the foot is easily infected and what may have been only a minor discomfort may become a major problem. All blisters should be treated with care. Foot services in the presence of friction blisters should not be provided. Counsel the client about shoes and skin products to help prevent blisters from occurring. Provide foot services only after the blister is totally healed. If the blister is infected or appears too severe for the client to care for himself refer him to a podiatrist or physician.

Blisters From Other Causes

Burns, chemical irritants, fungal infections, bacterial infections, and many other internal or external causes may produce skin blisters. Some pressure sores, particularly on the heel, start as a simple blister on the skin. It is important to be able to determine the cause of the blister to give proper care. If there is the slightest suspicion that a blister you observe is anything other than a friction blister, refer the client to a podiatrist or physician. Without treatment of the primary cause the condition may become more severe.

Callus

Calluses (**tyloma**) are biomechanically induced conditions that occur mainly on the sole or edges of the foot. They may also occur on other areas of the foot where excessive intermittent friction and rubbing occur with any regularity. The callus usually extends an enlarged area of irritated skin and its edges blend into the normal surrounding skin. The classical friction callus is seen under the ball of the foot (Figure 4-5). Calluses are the result of long-term abnormal stresses on the skin. This is in contrast to blisters, which form after short-term excessive stress to the affected area of skin. The skin does not have time to produce the extra keratin to protect itself and as a result a blister forms instead of a callus.

——— **L.O. 7**

The formation of callus is the skin's attempt to protect itself from excessive irritation or mechanical stresses. An abnormal gait pattern will result in extra shearing or friction forces being applied to the bottom of the foot. The intermittent force of this abnormal walking causes the basal cell layer of the skin to produce extra keratin. This results in the thickening of the skin in the area of irritation. The yellow discoloration of the callus is due to the extra keratin within the tissue.

The symptom of a callus is usually a burning type of pain. Other symptoms vary from a throbbing ache to a sharp stabbing pain. These symptoms depend on the location

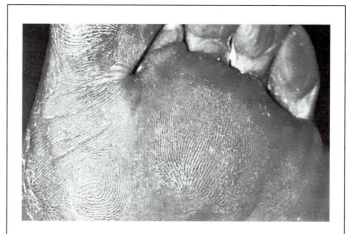

Figure 4-5 Classic friction callus on the ball of the foot

and thickness of the callus. The nail professional may attempt to remove callus tissue with the foot files or sloughing creams developed for this purpose. WARNING: The use of Credo® blades or other sharp instruments is not advisable. In most states it is illegal for the nail professional to use a sharp instrument to remove callus tissue. It takes extra training, skill, and years of practice to develop the dexterity and feel of just how much callus to remove without causing injury. If the callus is too thick to be adequately reduced with the foot file or abrasive creams the client should be referred to the podiatrist for proper reduction of the callus. The podiatrist will also determine the cause of the callus and will be able to recommend treatment to possibly prevent a recurrence of the problem. Follow-up foot services by the nail professional are then indicated.

Intractable Plantar Keratoma (IPK). This callus is differentiated from a shearing or friction callus in that it has a deep "core" within it. It is a common misconception that this "core" is the "root" of the callus. The word root implies that the callus is a living structure. This is far from the truth! Many over-the-counter callus medications are sold as being able to "get out the root." This implies a cure and much money has been made from this misconceived idea.

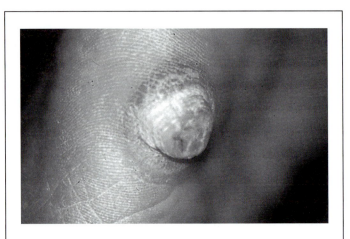

Figure 4-6 Example of an intractable plantar keratoma under the fifth metatarsal head. It almost appears as a horn on the bottom of the foot. The edges are well defined.

The typical IPK is found under a single weight-bearing area, usually under one of the metatarsal heads (Figure 4-6). The edges of the IPK are well demarcated and do not blend into the surrounding normal tissues. The center of the lesion is quite deep and called the "central area of irritation." This is the area where the most pressure or irritation is present. Because of this more callus is formed at this point. The pressure of walking causes this area to be pressed deep into the skin. This results in more irritation and the formation of more callus forcing the callus deeper into the skin. The edges around the IPK become irritated but not to the extent of the "central area of irritation." The resultant IPK is shaped like a pyramid with the top of the pyramid being the "central area of irritation." Clients with an IPK should be referred to the podiatrist for treatment.

Heel Callus. Some people form large amounts of callus tissue around their heels (Figure 4-7). As the callus builds up, cracks or

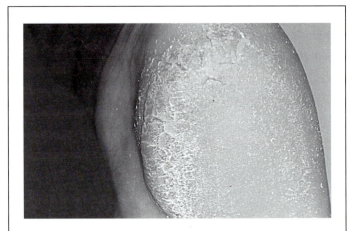

Figure 4-7 A heel callus. Some get much worse than this.

fissures form along the lines of stress in the skin. These cracks may extend down into the underlying normal tissues and become painful or infected. The cause in many cases is not known. In others abnormal biomechanical stresses on the tissues surrounding the heel is the cause. Shoes that do not support the heel properly can be a contributing factor. Certain fungal infections may also be a causative factor. Whatever the cause, this condition can be unsightly and painful.

The nail professional should not attempt to care for callused heels if the fissures are deep and extend into the normal tissues. Clients with extremely thick heel calluses should be referred to the podiatrist for reduction of the callus. If the podiatrist finds that the condition is caused or aggravated by a fungus, treatment for this can be prescribed. Follow-up pedicures to keep the callus under control are then indicated.

Products such as Tropical Harmony™ and Bag Balm™ may help control this problem. One must stress to the client that these products will not cure the problem but with their continual use and routine pedicures they will be able to control it. Clients must be willing to help in the care of their heels at home; otherwise all you do will not be enough to relieve the condition.

Clients with heel calluses may need referral to a podiatrist.

Corns (Heloma, Clavus)

When people say they have a "corn," think of a callus on the toe. This is because a corn is really a callus. There is no real difference other than positional. The causes of corns and calluses are the same—friction and pressure. Corns on the sides or top of the toes in most cases are caused by improperly fit shoes rubbing on a bony prominence on the toe. Corns on the ends of the toes are usually the result of a malposition of the toe. This causes the tip of the toe to be a weight-bearing point during walking. The extra pressure and friction on this usually non-weight-bearing area during walking results in the buildup of painful callus.

Some corns have a deep core often termed the "root or seed." This condition is again the result of a "central area of irritation" causing more callus to build up in one area. Mechanical stress and shoe pressure force the callus into the skin in the same manner as described for the IPK. The main thing to stress to clients is that corns are not alive and they do not have a "root or seed," which if removed will cure them. Corns are nature's way of trying to protect the skin; however, when they become too thick from the irritation on the area they then become painful.

Corns may be divided into two categories: hard corns (heloma durum) and soft corns (heloma molle). Hard corns are on the tops and ends of the toes (Figure 4-8). They are usually yellowish in color and have a very hard texture. Soft corns are found in between or deep in the web spaces between the toes (Figure 4-9). Their cause is the same as a hard corn—

——— L.O. 8

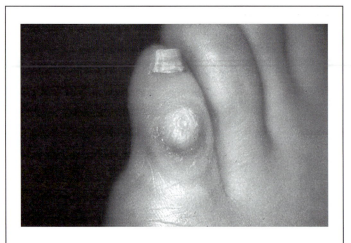

Figure 4-8 *A typical hard corn on the side of the fifth toe*

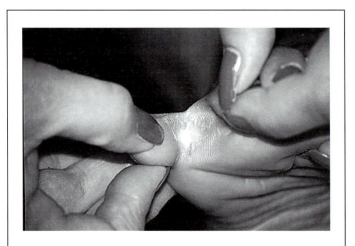

Figure 4-9 *A soft corn in the web space between the fourth and fifth toes. It has a white spongy appearance and is often misdiagnosed as a fungus.*

pressure and friction. They are termed soft because they develop a whitish color and have a spongy texture because of the wetness of the perspiration found between the toes. Because of their location, soft corns are more prone to infection and ulceration. Soft corns are also often misdiagnosed as fungal infections between the toes. Listen to your clients: If they complain of pain between their toes the problem in most instances will be a soft corn. Fungal infections between the toes generally are not painful unless they are secondarily infected by a bacterium.

The permanent treatment of a corn can be as simple as recommending a properly fit shoe. In the podiatrist's office simple surgical straightening of the toe or the removal of the bony bump will "cure" the corn. WARNING: DO NOT recommend the use of medicated pads or liquids for the home treatment of corns or calluses. These over-the-counter treatments all have an acid base, which in theory softens and eats away the callus tissue. The problem is that they are hard to keep only on the corn or callus. They also do not know when to stop working and can easily result in an acid burn to the underlying skin. This results in an opening for infection and more pain and disability.

The nail professional should only attempt to remove hard corns in a similar manner as was discussed for the removal of callus tissue. Do not use sharp cutting instruments for the removal of corns. If you cannot remove enough callus in the recommended manner to make your clients comfortable, refer them to the podiatrist for proper care and treatment of the problem. The removal of callus from a soft corn, because of the possibility of infection and ulceration, should be preformed only by the podiatrist.

Wart (Verruca, Papilloma, Plantar Wart)

Warts on the foot as in other areas of the body are caused by the papovavirus. They are true tumors of the skin in that they do not extend below the basal cell layer. It is thought that the virus enters the skin directly through areas that are subject to trauma. Shoe trauma and pressure traumas on the

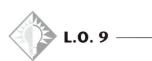

L.O. 9

bottom of the foot most probably increase the incidence of warts on the feet. Warts caused by a virus are in theory transmittable from one person to another, but this is rare.

Warts on the foot, particularly on the bottom of the foot, can be difficult to distinguish from calluses. If they are on a weight-bearing area they cause more pressure and irritation in that area, thus more callus is formed covering the wart. If they are under a direct weight-bearing area, such as under a metatarsal head, they appear much like an IPK. In these areas they are very painful when walking (as are IPKs). Eighty to 90% of what people think are warts on the bottom of their feet are really calluses. Warts between the toes can have the appearance of a soft corn in that they become white and have a spongy appearance. In non-weight-bearing areas, such as the top of the foot, warts have a similar appearance as warts on other areas of the body. Mosaic warts are so called because they resemble the appearance of a mosaic tile floor. A mosaic wart is composed of many individual warts compressed tightly together. The name **plantar wart** merely tells us the location of the wart—the plantar surface or sole of the foot.

When warts first appear the individual will think he has stepped on a piece of glass or a splinter, and will generally try to "remove" the offending object, usually with a needle. This seems to cause the wart to become larger or even to spread. The reason the individual thinks he has stepped on something is that warts have small capillaries within them. A capillary seen in the wart has the appearance of a splinter, thus the misconception of a foreign body as being the cause of the discomfort (Figure 4-10).

Warts are not caused by a foreign object embedded in the foot.

There are many different treatments for warts. This tells us that all of the treatments work sometimes but none work all the time. Some warts will spontaneously disappear. Others persist and require medical treatment to remove them. Treatments vary from hypnotherapy to actual surgical excision. There has been fairly good success with the application of various acids to the warts. There is no specific time period for treating a wart. They may be treated once or many times before the warts are gone. One particular case was a lady who presented with at least 20 individual warts scattered about her foot. Where to start her treatment? She had five warts under the free edge of her big toenail that were bothering her the most. These were removed surgically to cause

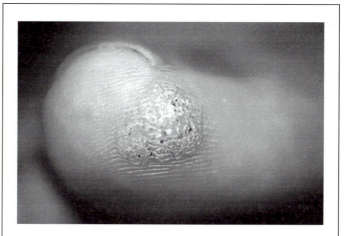

Figure 4-10 *This is a group of warts on the side of the big toe but they may occur anyplace on the foot. Notice the small black dots often mistaken for a sliver of wood. On the bottom of the foot these warts would be covered with a thick layer of callus.*

the least injury to the nail. By the time this area was healed, approximately three weeks, all the rest of the warts had spontaneously disappeared!

The nail professional should not be afraid to perform a foot service on a client with a wart. The probability of catching the wart is remote. Do not attempt to remove the callus from over the wart. If you are filing a callus and see small black dots or small points of bleeding you have probably been removing callus from over a wart. Warts bleed; properly reduced calluses do not. You should refer the client with a wart to a podiatrist or dermatologist for care. Because warts have a tendency to multiply and also become more resistant to treatment the longer they are present, early treatment of this condition should be encouraged.

Plantar Porokeratosis

These are small circular lesions found on the plantar surface of the foot. They have a deep core or plug of callus in the center. They can be found in full weight-bearing areas such as under the metatarsal heads or in non-weight-bearing areas such as in the longitudinal arch. They are hard to distinguish from a wart. Depending on their location they can be quite painful to walk on.

Studies have related the causative factor as being a plugged sweat gland. It has been theorized that the duct of the gland becomes plugged because of pressure. This results in further irritation and callus formation within the duct. The callus may in some cases be easily picked out of the area thus relieving some of the pressure. If the lesion is too painful refer the client to a podiatrist who can remove the callus plug. Some cases require actual surgical excision to relieve them on a permanent basis.

Fungal Infections of the Skin

Skin fungal infections include **tinea pedis**, **dermatophytosis**, **athlete's foot**, and **ringworm**. More than 100,000 known species of fungi are present in nature! Of this vast group of fungi only about 175 live on or in the human body. Of these 175, under normal conditions, only about 20 cause systemic disease to develop within the body. **Yeasts** and **molds** also fall within the classification of fungi. Some of the infections caused by these fungi are referred to as "tinea" infections. This word comes from the Latin word for worm and is used because of the worm-like appearance of the advancing edges of the infection. From this comes the common term "ringworm" used to describe many fungal infections of the skin.

Fungi form **spores**, which have a hard outer coating like an egg. Under proper circumstances when a spore comes in contact with the skin it will **germinate** within 4 to 6 hours and cause an infection. Intact healthy skin is a good barrier against fungal infections. In addition, the normal dry-

Of the thousands of known species of fungi, only about 20 cause disease in humans.

ness of the skin inhibits the growth of fungi, particularly the **Candida** (yeast, **monilia**) species, which is always with us.

Fungal infections of the skin may be acquired from contact with infected persons or from their clothes, from the soil, or from an infected pet. Others that normally live on the human body may cause infection when resistance is lowered because of injuries or other disease processes. Fungi are opportunistic and will take advantage of any weakness that allows them to grow. Candida is a prime example of this process. It is always present on and within our body and is quick to overgrow and cause infection when resistance is reduced.

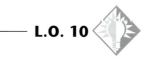

Tinea infections account for about one-third of the skin problems seen in the foot. The majority of the fungal infections of the feet are caused by only three different fungi: *Trichophyton rubrum, Trichophyton mentagrophytes,* and *Epidermophyton floccosum.* All of these fungi are found as spores in nature, which under the right conditions will cause infection. Proper conditions are a warm, moist, and dark environment. Because we wear hosiery and shoes that create this set of circumstances, the fungus has a perfect opportunity to grow. Footgear is then one of the major contributing factors of tinea pedis.

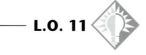

Another contributing factor is the susceptibility of the individual. Some people have a natural resistance and others do not. Consider the husband and wife who are married for 50 years. The husband has had tinea pedis for most of their married life, but his wife has never had the infection. The only explanation can be that she is not susceptible to the fungus. Physical **debilitation** also increases a person's susceptibility to this condition. Poor circulation, diabetes, and other systemic diseases all lower the body's resistance to fungal infections. Elderly individuals who lose the elasticity in their skin or those whose skin becomes dry and cracked are also susceptible to fungal infections of the feet.

Fungal infections on the foot are generally seen as two distinct types. One is a dry scaly form called chronic **hyperkeratotic** tinea pedis. The second is a more acute form called acute inflammatory tinea pedis. The hyperkeratotic form is characterized by a dry scaly formation on the skin. The edges of the scaly areas are usually slightly inflamed and red. Itching may or may not be present. The soles and sides of the feet are usually involved in a moccasin-like distribution (Figure 4-11). *Tinea*

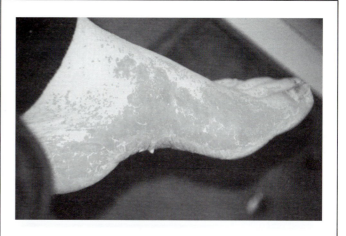

Figure 4-11 Chronic hyperkeratotic form of tinea pedis in the typical moccasin-like pattern

rubrum is the usual causative organism of the chronic hyperkeratotic form of tinea pedis. It is not unusual for an individual to have this type of tinea only on one foot. On occasion, if the hand is also infected only one may be involved. This condition may persist in this pattern for years. There is no explanation as to why this happens.

The acute inflammatory form is characterized by blisters (large or small) that may break and ooze. Itching is present, the skin may crack and become soft in the infected area. With the openings in the skin it is not uncommon for a secondary bacterial infection to start. One of the first areas in which this form of fungus usually occurs is between the fourth and fifth toes. The skin becomes whitish and a painful fissure may occur deep between the toes. (This condition is hard to distinguish from a soft corn in the same area.) This is the typical form of tinea pedis we think of as "athlete's foot." The causative organism is generally *T. mentagrophytes* although *E. floccosum* may at times be the primary cause of this acute form.

Candida, also known as monilia or yeast, needs a warm moist environment to cause infection. The area between the toes, particularly the fourth and fifth is most often involved with this organism. The skin between the toes becomes whitish and cracked. Areas of the outer skin will slough off leaving a bright red inflamed area underneath. In some cases this infection will also involve the nails and the soft tissues around the nail. The nail will have a typical spongy yellowish color and become loose from the underlying nail bed. When the nail is trimmed away the bed will be red and moist. The soft tissue around the nail will be puffy and inflamed. Medical treatment is necessary in these advanced candida infections.

In some cases during an acute episode of a tinea infection small blisters may appear on the sides of the fingers. This process is called an "id reaction." This process does not represent a true fungal infection in the hand because no fungus can be cultured from the blisters. The blisters are a hypersensitive reaction to the fungal infection in another part of the body. When the primary infection is cured the reaction in the hand will resolve by itself without direct treatment. This is an interesting phenomenon and one that should be recognized by the nail professional.

The nail professional need not be afraid to give foot services to an individual who has the chronic hyperkeratotic type of fungal infection on the feet. Latex examination gloves during the service are a good precaution particularly if there is an open cut or injury on the hands of the nail professional. The actual risk of transmitting this infection to the person giving the service is minimal. The simple act of washing the hands after the service is the main preventive measure needed to stop cross-infections. The use of proper sanitization procedures within the salon (see Chapter 9) will reduce the risk of

Proper and careful salon hygiene will help prevent infections.

transmission to acceptable levels. Remember the fungus that causes this infection likes a warm, moist, dark environment in which to grow. The hands do not generally meet these conditions.

The acute inflammatory form of tinea pedis should be approached with caution by the nail professional. An acute infection with weeping open blisters should not be serviced. An early or very mild infection, such as is often seen between the fourth and fifth toes, could receive a foot service using the precautions mentioned in the previous paragraph. Again it must be stressed that proper sanitization practices be used to prevent cross-contamination infections from occurring.

There are over-the-counter antifungal medications that the nail professional may recommend for mild tinea infections of the foot. Lotrimin® and Tinactin® are two that were previously only obtainable through a doctor's prescription. They are excellent for many of the milder forms of fungal infections of the foot. Lotrimin®, in particular, is recommended for the *Candida* or yeast infections seen between the toes. Advise the client to use the product for at least three to four weeks. It will take that long to destroy the fungus even though the itching and scaling will stop much sooner. For the resistant or the more involved fungal infections of the foot, the nail professional should refer the client to a podiatrist or dermatologist for treatment.

Refer to the medical specialist those clients who have acute or long-standing fungal infections.

FOOT NOTES

There are more than 100,000 known species of fungus! The vast majority of these do not cause infections in humans. Many fungi are present on or in the human body but under normal circumstances do not cause infections. The environment created on the foot because of shoes and hosiery is an excellent area for fungi to grow. At least one-third of the skin conditions seen on the foot are caused by fungi.

The two main types of fungal infections seen on the foot are the chronic hyperkeratotic and the acute inflammatory forms. The nail professional may give foot services to individuals who have these infections as described. Proper sanitation and protective measures are a must when providing these services! Make recommendations for home treatments for the minor fungal infections and refer to the medical specialist those clients who have acute or long-standing fungal infections.

Bacterial Infections of the Foot

L.O. 12

Bacteria are normal inhabitants on and within the human body. When given the opportunity and the proper set of circumstances, bacteria will cause infection. Bacteria need a **portal of entry** or opening through the skin to enable them to multiply in the numbers necessary to create disease. The warm moist environment on the foot is an excellent area for bacteria to live. A portal of entry is all that is needed to complete the circumstance for an infection.

Just as we find certain animals living in particular environments in nature so do we find certain bacteria living in or on particular areas of our body. Bacterial species of *Staphylococcus*, *Streptococcus*, and *Pseudomonas* are the predominant bacteria found on the foot. Most of the infections on the foot are caused by these organisms. *Staphylococcus aureus* is the usual infective organism associated with ingrown toenails. A localized infection with yellow-colored pus is typically seen with this organism. Infections in the skin and other areas of the foot are generally caused by *Streptococcus* species; however, in most foot infections, they do not form pus pockets or **abscesses**. These infections are usually seen as swollen red areas within or under the skin with an ill-defined border or margin. They spread throughout the soft tissues and in the foot are most often the causative organism of the "red streak" seen up the foot and leg, which in reality is an inflamed lymph vessel. *Pseudomonas* species prefer a more moist environment so are mainly found between the toes and along nail borders or under a loose nail. *Pseudomonas* species are resistant to many antibiotics. Because of this, long-term chronic infections of the nails or web spaces are commonly associated with this organism. A greenish or bluish discoloration of the infected tissues is often seen with a *Pseudomonas* infection.

The foot, because of the many different bacteria that are present on it, is a common site for mixed infections.

Once an infection has started other infectious bacteria will become involved in the process. This then is called a "mixed" infection in which more than one bacterium is involved. This complicates the treatment of the infection because of the resistance of some bacteria to certain antibiotics. In the treatment of severe mixed infections it is not uncommon to see two or more antibiotics being used at the same time. The foot, because of the many different bacteria that are present on it, is a common site for mixed infections.

Poor hygiene, physical debilitation, or anything that lowers the resistance of an individual are contributing factors to the severity of an infective process. Those with diabetes or arteriosclerosis are prime examples of this. The elderly and people with dry, cracked skin are also prone to infection. Nail professionals must be knowledgeable about the status of each client to reduce the risks of infection caused by their services. Good sanitation practices are a must. Care should always be taken not to create a portal of entry for the infective process to begin. If during a service a cut or abrasion of the skin is created do not disregard it! Inform the client what has happened. Apply a disinfectant such as alcohol and an antibiotic ointment with an adhesive dressing. Tell the client to call you if she has any problem. If a problem develops see that the client receives proper medical attention.

Many patients with minor infections of the nails will say they thought the pedicurist had cut them during a service. They are usually upset because they perceive the pedicurist/manicurist did not know what she was doing. This situation in most cases would not arise if the nail professional had handled the client in a professional manner. Sooner or later in your career you will cause a client to bleed. This is part of the risk you assume when you become a licensed nail professional! When it happens, handle the incident professionally and the risk of an infection will be dramatically reduced. Your client will also gain a greater respect for your abilities.

If you accidentally cut a client, handle the matter professionally to reduce the risk of infection.

Learn to recognize the signs and symptoms of infections (redness, heat, swelling, and pain) and when seen counsel the client and refer for proper medical attention. When the skin is cracked or dry recommend skin care products that will help the condition. Cracks or fissures between the toes are common. Recommend the use of antiseptic or antifungal powders to dry and heal the area before infections start. Your clients are placing their trust in your abilities. It is your responsibility to advise, counsel and, if necessary, refer them for more intensive care if the problem is beyond your expertise.

Hyperhidrosis

Hyperhidrosis is a condition of excessive perspiration formation. It is estimated that about 25% of the population are affected by this problem. There is no predisposition between the sexes. The affected areas are usually the palms of the hands and the soles of the feet. Some cases of hyperhidrosis have no identifiable cause. It is thought to be hereditary. Other cases of this condition can be directly related to specific causes such as diabetes, fevers, anemias, hyperthyroidism, and in rare instances tumors of the nervous system.

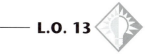 **L.O. 13**

Eccrine sweat glands produce the perspiration. Because the sole of the foot has only sweat glands, and no sebaceous glands, the condition is most noticeable in this area. It has been estimated that there are over 600 eccrine sweat glands per square centimeter on the soles of the feet. If all of these are actively working at the same time copious amounts of perspiration are produced. There was one male patient who would sit in the treatment chair and the sweat would literally run off of his heels while being treated. His hands and underarms were the same. He was extremely embarrassed about this condition and had been to many doctors for it. All treatments had been unsuccessful. He was an extremely nervous individual which seemed to add to the problem. There were no answers for him other than the usual powders and hygiene recommendations that he was already using.

With this condition the skin between the toes and on the sole is whitish and spongy looking. The surrounding areas of skin are usually pinker than normal, appearing inflamed, but are cool to the touch. Some individuals with hyperhidrosis will have symptoms of itching or burning and may even form small water blisters within the skin.

Bromhidrosis

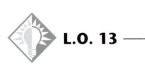

L.O. 13

This term refers to sweat having an obnoxious odor. Normal sweat is composed of water, potassium and chloride salts, lactate, and urea. It usually has no odor. In the presence of excessive perspiration the bacteria on the foot begin to overgrow and decompose the normal protein debris on the surface of the skin. The breakdown chemicals and gases formed in this process produce the foul smell associated with this condition. Just as different strains of bacteria are used in the production of Limburger and Brie cheeses, which have totally different smells, the different species of bacteria present on the foot account for the particular odor produced.

Scrupulous hygiene is necessary to reduce the numbers of bacteria present on the foot. The daily use of surgical soaps will help. The main thrust of care must be directed at reducing the amount of perspiration being formed. Cotton socks changed several times daily depending on the severity of the condition will help keep the foot drier. Highly absorbant powders such as Zeasorb AF® will also help. Antiperspirants sprayed on the feet morning and evening can be helpful. In severe cases the use of an electrical stimulating device called the Drionic® produced by General Medical Company of Los Angeles is said to be of help. Doctors can prescribe certain drugs that act on the autonomic nervous system and in some cases will help reduce the formation of sweat. The problem with this is that the drug will affect the entire body and may produce adverse side effects. In high strung and nervous individuals, relaxation techniques or biofeedback training may be beneficial.

Perspiration can be a clue to various body problems.

As a nail professional you should be well versed in this condition and be able to discuss it with your affected client. Routine pedicures will help the client with foot hygiene as well as be extremely relaxing. Recommend products that will reduce the production of perspiration as well as assist the client in keeping the feet drier during the day. This client will appreciate anything that you can do to help with this embarrassing condition.

Anhidrosis

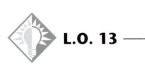

L.O. 13

Anhidrosis means the inability to produce sweat. In the foot it may be a localized process or part of a generalized condition. Skin conditions such as contact, **atopic**, and **exfoliative** dermatitis may cause this condition.

Diabetes, heavy metal poisoning, certain malignancies, some kidney diseases, and **cirrhosis** of the liver also may be a cause. Localized conditions such as injury to the foot, decreased blood supply as in arteriosclerosis, tumors that affect the nerves to the lower extremity, and a congenital absence of the sweat glands all can be causative factors.

The skin is dry, scaly, and parchment like. Painful fissures or cracks may develop. The nail professional should recommend hydrating creams and lotions for this problem if the skin is intact. Urea-based or vitamin A-based products that hydrate seem to be the most beneficial. If the problem is severe refer the client for medical evaluation by a dermatologist or podiatrist.

Contact Dermatitis

This condition is caused by the skin coming into contact with an irritating agent that causes inflammation. There are two different types of contact dermatitis—primary and secondary. Primary irritants include over-the-counter corn medications or other toxic substances that will cause irritation to the skin of every individual who comes into contact with the substance. Secondary contact dermatitis is an individual's allergic reaction to a specific substance or chemical. The classic secondary type seen in the foot is caused by the chemicals used in tanning leather. The skin will be irritated in a specific pattern where the leather comes into contact with the skin (Figure 4-12).

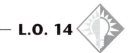

The care of this condition is like a game of 20 questions. Identifying the irritant is the key to curing the problem, but sometimes this is difficult. A patient had an allergy to rubber products. She had an irritation on the bottoms of both feet when she was first seen. It had the typical appearance of athlete's foot. Cultures were negative and treatment did not help the condition. It was finally determined that the orthotics she had been wearing had a covering that had been glued in place with rubber cement. The perspiration from her feet was leaching the irritant through the top cover of the orthotic and causing the dermatitis. When she discontinued wearing those orthotics the skin irritation disappeared.

Piezogenic Papules

This is an interesting finding on the heels of some people. It causes no problem but may be alarming to the client. Papules appear as small yellowish bumps around the medial and lateral aspect of the heel (Figure 4-13). They are most noticeable when standing. The bumps are small

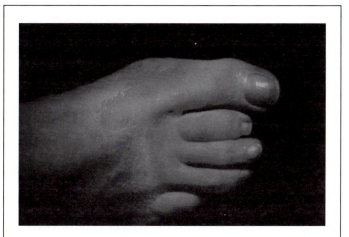

Figure 4-12 *Contact dermatitis caused by the chemicals used in tanning the leather in the patients shoes. Notice that the red area over the top of the toes and foot is only where the leather contacted the skin.*

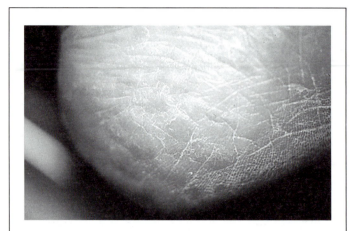

Figure 4-13 Notice the small colored bumps on the skin of this heel. These are piezogenic papules. They appear in this picture because the patient is not standing on her feet.

extrusions of subcutaneous fat through defects in the underlying tissues. When no weight is on the foot they are difficult to see and if present at all they have the coloring of the skin. They are usually not painful and are most often seen in young active individuals who have little extra subcutaneous fat. On occasion in obese individuals the papules may become painful after prolonged standing. A supportive heel protector will usually help if symptoms are present.

Cold Injuries to the Foot

Chilblain (Pernio). This is one of the mildest forms of cold injury. It generally involves the toes. It appears as reddish purple blotches on the skin that burn, sting, and itch. In more severe cases there may be blister or ulcer formation, seen mainly in diabetic and arteriosclerotic patients. In theory, however, it may occur in anyone who may have a sensitivity to cold. It does not take freezing cold to produce this condition. In Sacramento, the climate is relatively mild but after a prolonged period of dampness and fog with temperatures in the 30s and low 40s we begin to see this problem.

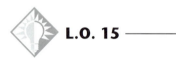
L.O. 15

Severe cases require medical care. In mild forms the client must be advised to wear warm footgear during the cold weather. Another recommendation is to wrap lambs' wool around the toes before putting on hosiery. This gives added warmth to the toes. Affected individuals will always need to be careful during cold weather because once they have had the problem they will be more susceptible to it in the future.

L.O. 15

Frostbite. This is the actual freezing of tissues. The extremities, particularly the feet, are susceptible to frostbite. Superficial frostbite affects the skin and subcutaneous tissues. Deep or severe frostbite affects the tendons, muscles, and in some cases the bone. The superficial form appears as a white patch of frozen skin. The area will usually heal in a few days without any permanent damage to the tissues. The severe form results in the death of tissues. The area affected and the depth of the freezing will dictate the necessary treatment. This may be surgical **debridement** of the dead tissues or possibly even amputation depending on the severity of the injury.

Pigmented Nevus (Mole)

L.O. 16

The pigmented **nevus** or mole is the most common "tumor" of the skin. They appear in childhood and also in adulthood. In the early stages they appear as nonraised tan or brownish areas on the skin. As they mature they may become raised and will exhibit many varying sizes, shapes, surfaces, and colors ranging from tan to dark brown (Figure 4-14). They will have a defined margin and in some cases will even have hair growing out of them. Most pigmented nevi do not cause a problem and there is no need for them to be removed. Nevi on the palms of the hands and the soles of the feet seem to have a higher incidence of becoming malignant than those in other areas of the body. Some medical specialists advocate the removal of all nevi in these areas because of this, whereas the majority opinion now is to watch for changes before excision. Studies have shown predictable changes that will occur if a nevus is exhibiting malignant tendencies.

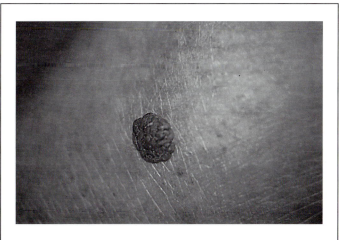

Figure 4-14 *This is a raised nevus. This one appears as a small berry and is reddish to brown in color. They come in all sizes and colors. Nevi should be watched closely for any changes in appearance which may indicate an early beginning of a malignant melanoma.*

As a nail professional you will have occasion to observe nevi on the extremities. The main thing is to discuss the presence of the nevus with the client. Most patients are well aware of their presence and somewhat knowledgeable about the possibility of them becoming malignant. You should advise them to seek a medical opinion if they notice a change in color or size in the nevus. Also medical attention should be sought for nevi that have not been injured but which bleed, ooze, or ulcerate. If you have any question or suspicion about a nevus you should strongly recommend a consultation with a dermatologist. Early detection of malignant changes within a nevus will save a life.

Melanoma

A **melanoma** is a cancer of the pigment-producing cells of the skin (Figure 4-15). It is the most serious malignancy of the skin and if left untreated will spread throughout the body and cause death. A complete cure of this disease depends on early detection and subsequent surgical excision. This condition may arise from a nonmalignant pigmented nevus or from pigment cells within normally appearing skin. Its cause is unknown. However, an association with the exposure to ultraviolet light may be a contributing factor.

Approximately 1% of the cancers diagnosed in the United States are melanomas. Of

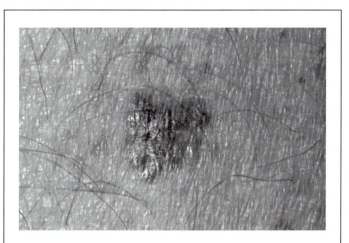

Figure 4-15 *Melanoma of the skin. Notice the irregular borders around the lesion. It is not totally black but has black, brown, and reddish colors in it. Refer any nevus that has these borders or that you or the client is suspicous of to the dermatologist.*

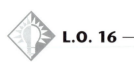

L.O. 16 ———— those diagnosed melanomas, some 30% to 40% occur on the lower extremity. Melanomas are usually quite dark in color but can range from a brownish to reddish colors. The **amelanotic** melanoma appears as a red moist tumor-like structure on the skin. The margins of the melanoma are uneven and tend to blend into the surrounding tissues. In some cases on the palms and soles they may mimic the appearance of a wart. As a nail professional you must be on the lookout for any suspicious pigmented lesions of the skin. Know what to look for as we have discussed in the pigmented nevus section and here. Advise your clients about the subject of melanomas and refer any questionable or suspicious lesions to a dermatologist for evaluation.

Psoriasis

L.O. 17 ———— **Psoriasis** is a generalized disease that also may produce mild to severe effects on the foot (Figure 4-16). The actual cause of psoriasis is unknown. In affected individuals the time required for the basal cells to reach the epithelial layer of the skin (epidermal turnover time) is extremely short. Normally it takes 28 to 30 days for this process, whereas in the psoriatic individual this time is reduced to 3 or 4 days. This extremely active turnover time of the skin cells produces the typical silvery scaly plaques of skin seen with this disease. On removal of the scale the underlying skin will appear red and inflamed because of the dilated capillaries underlying the area. There may also be some pinpoint bleeding from the capillaries in the area after the scale is removed.

There are many forms of psoriasis. Those seen most commonly in the lower extremity include silvery plaque lesions, pustular psoriasis, and psoriatic **keratoderma** of the sole of the foot and the palm of the hand. **Interdigital** psoriasis, also known as "white psoriasis" (rare), psoriasis of the nails (to be discussed in another chapter), and psoriatic arthritis (see Chapter 4) are also seen in the feet. All of these forms may vary from mild to severe. The plaque form is the type generally seen on other areas of the body. The pustular form is first seen on the soles as small sterile blisters of pus that dry as dark brownish crusts before peeling off. As this form progresses the entire sole may be involved, with the skin between the blisters having the silvery scaly appearance of psoriasis. In the keratoderma form massive amounts of yellowish or grayish callus-like tissues are formed. Deep painful fissures are generally present. This and the pustular forms may be so severe as to cause the indi-

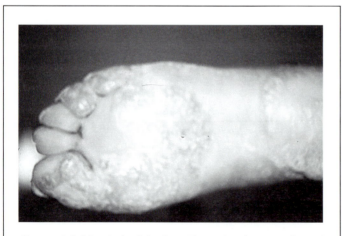

Figure 4-16 Psoriasis of the feet. The entire plantar surface of both feet is involved, with large amounts of callus buildup, particularly on the heels. The palmar surfaces of both hands are also involved in the same manner.

vidual great pain during walking. The interdigital or white form appears as white macerated tissue in the web spaces between the toes. It is hard to distinguish this form from a fungal infection and a surgical biopsy of the tissue in most cases is the only way to arrive at a definitive diagnosis.

As a nail professional you will see some forms of psoriasis during your career. Consult with the client's dermatologist or podiatrist before doing a foot service. The skin of a person with psoriasis is fragile and any injury no matter how slight may cause an extension of the psoriatic lesions.

DEFORMITIES OF THE FOOT

This section discusses some common deformities seen in the foot. Unless there are any open sores or ulcerations associated with these conditions, foot services may be performed by the nail professional. In most of these cases a pedicure with warm water baths and a good massage will be beneficial for the client.

Arch Deformities

Flat Foot (Pes Planus). Much has been written about the arches of the foot. We are all acquainted with the "flat foot." Our mothers all worried about our feet and bought our shoes so they would have a good arch support so that we would not get "flat feet." Little did they realize that we inherited our feet from her and dad and that no matter what shoes we wore if we were born to have flat feet we would have them! As we have already discussed in the gait cycle section of this chapter what is generally referred to as a flat foot is in reality a pronated foot that we are born with.

— L.O. 18

Foot deformities require special attention and care.

A true flat foot (one we are born with) is rare. The true flat foot has no longitudinal arch in either the non-weight-bearing or weight-bearing state. The bones and soft tissues are meant to be in that position from the first moment of conception. The true flat foot is a stable foot and will not be painful. It does not need an arch support; in fact, an arch support would in most cases be quite painful.

The pronated flat foot is another story as we have seen. In this foot there is an arch present when the foot is in a non-weight-bearing status. However, when body weight is applied to the foot, the arch appears to flatten out. In old age, because of the abnormal stresses placed on the foot, many arthritic changes occur in the joints of the foot and a rigid flat foot is the result. The longitudinal arch is absent in both the non-weight-bearing and the weight-bearing conditions and there is no longer any motion within the majority of the joints of the foot. The pronated flat foot is one that causes many of the painful foot conditions we are discussing.

L.O. 18

High Arched Foot (Pes Cavus, Claw Foot). In this deformity of the longitudinal arch, the arch is extremely high. The foot is rigid and when the person stands the majority of the weight is on the heel and ball of the foot. The toes are dorsally contracted back on the metatarsal heads, presenting a clawed appearance. In some severe cases the ends of the toes do not even touch the ground when the foot is bearing weight.

This arch deformity may be hereditary or acquired. In the hereditary form the deformity can be traced back through the family. The acquired form is generally the result of neurologic disorders such as polio or **spina bifida** that causes muscle imbalances and contractures of the muscles within the foot as well as in the leg. The high arched foot is not comfortable to walk on and because of the high instep and contracted toes are very hard to fit into shoes. Corns on the toes may result from the **contractures** causing a rub on the shoe. Deep calluses may form under the metatarsal heads because of the extreme pressures being exerted on these areas. Because of the extra pressures on the instep a bony overgrowth may form, making it even harder to fit into shoes. An arch support or orthotic is beneficial in these cases. Severe cases may need custom made shoes or surgery to make them comfortable.

Digital Deformities

These are deformities relating to the toes. As a rule most of these deformities are caused by improper biomechanics of the pronated foot. Foot services may be done on clients with these deformities as long as no open sores or ulcerations are present. Reduce any calluses carefully with an abrasive file and sloughing creams. Refer acute conditions to the podiatrist for care. Many of these painful digital problems are easily fixed with some minor surgical procedures.

Hammertoe. This deformity is one of the most common deformities of the foot (Figure 4-17). In our society, because of shoes, the problem is usually painful. During the initial stages of formation of a hammertoe the tendons contract and hold the toe in the hammered position. The toe can be manually straightened but when released will return to the hammered position. This is termed a **flexible hammertoe**. As the deformity progresses

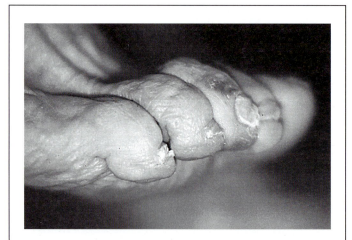

Figure 4-17 *Multiple hammertoes. The deformity is mainly at the proximal phalangeal joint with the toes taking on a C shape.*

arthritic changes occur within the joints of the toe and it becomes rigid. This then is termed a **rigid hammertoe**.

Hammertoes are generally seen in the second through fifth toes but may also occur in the great toe. The second toe seems to be affected more often than the other toes because of its greater length. The problem may be hereditary but is usually acquired as the result of improper biomechanics or shoes. Arthritis and muscular diseases also may cause this deformity. The majority of the deformity is at the proximal interphalangeal joint with the base of the intermediate phalanx being in a plantar flexed position in relation to the head of the proximal phalanx. This then forces a dorsiflexion of the proximal phalanx on the metatarsal and the distal phalanx becomes either flexed or extended on the intermediate phalanx. The end result of this deformity is that the top of the toe becomes elevated and begins rubbing on the shoe causing the formation of a corn. If the toe is flexed so that the tip comes into contact with the weight-bearing surface, a painful corn will form here also. If allowed to become thick, the corns will cause excessive pressure on the underlying tissues resulting in their breakdown. Infections of the toes are common because of this.

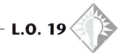
L.O. 19

Mallet Toe. A mallet toe is different from a hammertoe in that the deformity is at the distal interphalangeal joint (Figure 4-18). The distal phalanx is plantar flexed on the intermediate phalanx with the rest of the joints of the toe remaining in a relatively normal position. The result is a painful callus buildup on the tip of the toe that often breaks down and becomes infected. The causes of this deformity are the same as those for hammertoes.

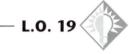
L.O. 19

The corns from these deformities usually result in pain and disability to the individual. A properly fit shoe with a deep toe box will help the symptoms. If the deformity is severe, particularly if it is fixed, a surgical correction will be required to give any permanent relief from the problem. The podiatrist can do this either in the office or in an outpatient surgical center. As a nail professional you may be able to relieve some of the pressure of the callus, in selected healthy clients, by filing it with a coarse file made for the purpose. Do not use the sharp cutting tools, often promoted as being safe, for this procedure. The risks and liabilities are too great. If sharp surgical trimming of the callus is necessary refer the client to a podiatrist for the procedure. For clients with less severe deformities you should discuss proper fitting and selection of shoes. Educate the

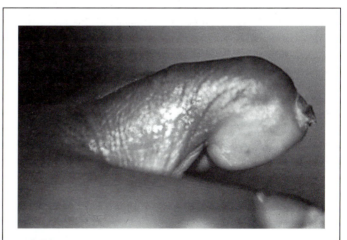

Figure 4-18 *Mallet toe. The deformity is at the distal phalangeal joint with the rest of the toe being relatively straight.*

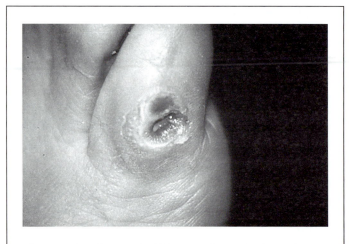

Figure 4-19 *Ulcer on the fifth toe as the result of a medicated corn pad. Note the complete loss of skin in the center of this ulcer.*

client about the problem. Recommend products such as Scholls™ lambs' wool, which will help pad the toes when wearing shoes, or Scholls Corn Cushions®. Do not recommend the products that have an adhesive backing that sticks to the skin because the adhesive itself will irritate the skin. Also clients will leave these products in place much too long, which also causes problems with the underlying skin. WARNING: NEVER recommend any of the products (liquids or disks) that have as their active ingredient salicylic or some other acid that is promoted as a corn or callus remover. These acid products are dangerous because they can cause burns and breakdowns of the underlying living skin (Figure 4-19). A podiatrist sees many infections and ulcers as a result of these acid-based products.

Congenital Overlapping Fifth Toe. This deformity consists of the toe overlapping over the fourth toe. In most cases it is not painful and causes little problem in shoes. In most instances this deformity is inherited. On occasion poorly fit shoes or muscle contractures after surgical reductions of hammertoe deformities may be a contributing factor. Improperly fit shoes, particularly pointed styles, may cause either a hard corn on the top of the toe or a soft corn between the fourth and fifth toes. This deformity also causes the fifth metatarsal head to be prominent where extra pressure from shoes may cause a callus to form. The prominent fifth metatarsal head is commonly called a tailor's bunion or bunionette (small bunion). The tailor's bunion may be present without the overlapping fifth toe. If this is the case, the cause is generally improper biomechanics of the foot. The symptoms (callus formation, pain in the area) are the result of shoe wear.

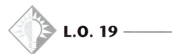 **L.O. 19** ──────

Properly fit shoes are very important. Discuss shoe fitting with these clients. Refer those with severe symptomatic deformities to the podiatrist for correction. The overlapping fifth toe is one foot condition in which a cosmetic correction is warranted for those who are embarrassed by it. In many instances a soft tissue correction will easily repair this problem.

L.O. 19 ──────

Hallux Valgus with Bunion. In this digital deformity the great toe points away from the midline of the body and the first metatarsal head becomes enlarged on the medial aspect of the foot (Figure 4-20). There have been many proposed causes of this condition but the primary cause is the biomechanical imbalance of the foot as the result of abnormal pronation. In rare instances the individual is born with the deformity. Inflammatory joint diseases such as rheumatoid arthritis can cause this condition. Shoes are an aggravating factor but only on infrequent occasions are they the actual cause.

The severity of the deformity does not seem to correspond with the symptoms. Some patients' hallux has been so deviated that the second toe was dislocated and overlapping the great toe. The only complaint from these patients was about pain in the second toe usually from a corn. Because of the dislocation at the second metatarsal phalangeal joint, a deep painful callus will form under the second metatarsal head on the bottom of the foot. As a nail professional see your role in the care of this problem as one of an educator. Discuss shoe fitting with your clients and advise them about the causes of the deviated toe. Care for the callus formation as has been previously described. Refer clients with symptoms to the podiatrist for more information and possible surgical correction of the deformity. The longer the symptoms are present the more destructive will be the changes taking place within the malpositioned joint resulting in the need for more complex surgery to repair it.

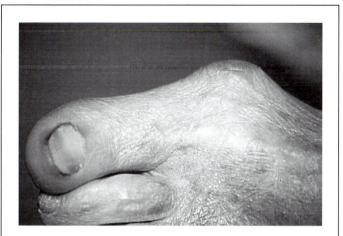

Figure 4-20 *Hallux valgus deformity of the great toe. The first metatarsal head becomes enlarged to form the bunion and the great toe deviates away from the midline of the body.*

MISCELLANEOUS FOOT DISORDERS

In this section we will discuss common foot disorders that the nail professional should be aware of. These conditions will not prevent the nail professional from providing a foot service. By being aware of them you will be able to counsel your client about the condition. You will also be able to make some general recommendations concerning the care necessary to relieve the problem.

Cold Feet

How many times have you heard a person say, "I know that I have poor circulation because my feet are always cold." The majority of the time cold feet do —— L.O. 20 not mean that the individual has poor circulation. It is rare that this condition represents a serious health problem. Remember from our previous discussion that one of the main functions of the skin is to control body temperature. This is accomplished by dilating or constricting the small surface blood vessels. This feeling of coldness in the feet in many cases is related to this process because the feet are richly supplied with small surface blood vessels.

Cold feet are usually nothing more than an uncomfortable nuisance.

Another common cause of cold feet is the evaporation of perspiration from the skin surface. The feet are well supplied with perspiration glands. As the perspiration evaporates heat is released. Individuals who perspire excessively are particularly prone to cold feet. Even under normal circumstances the evaporation of perspiration will cause the feet to feel cold. Stress will cause an individual to perspire excessively, and, therefore, may be a contributing factor to cold feet. Pathologic diseases that can contribute to cold feet include scleroderma, anemias, diabetes, peripheral vascular disease, and Raynaud's phenomenon. Some over-the-counter or prescription medications that cause **vasoconstriction** of the blood vessels will also contribute to this condition.

Nature will shunt blood to the vital organs such as the heart and brain at the expense of our hands and feet. Wearing warm clothes to keep the upper body warm will help to keep the feet warm. Exercise will also help this condition by causing the small blood vessels to dilate bringing more blood and warmth to the feet. Avoid nicotine and limit caffeine intake because both of these are vasoconstrictors. Reduce stress in daily life because high strung individuals seem to be more susceptible to the complaint of cold feet. Remember cold feet are usually nothing more than an uncomfortable nuisance. They are not generally the sign of some severe disease process.

Burning Feet

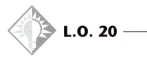 **L.O. 20**

This condition is not a primary foot problem. Burning sensations are carried over the pain nerve pathways. The condition of burning feet usually indicates an injury or irritation to the nerves in that area. It is characterized by complaints of generalized burning on the soles particularly at night. The sensations of burning may be so great as to cause the individual to sleep with the feet uncovered. The actual cause of the condition is many times unidentifiable. Nutritional deficiencies, such as lack of vitamin B12 as seen in pernicious anemia, are sometimes a cause. Alcoholics for the same reasons may present this condition. Because of the neuropathies associated with their disease, diabetics often have the complaint. Circulatory problems that result in a reduced blood supply to the nerves may also be a contributing factor to this uncomfortable condition.

For individuals who have no real identifiable disease processes that can be attributable to the cause of this condition, often recommended is a high potency vitamin B complex supplement as a trial treatment. The recommendation is one tablet in the morning and one at night and in some cases this will help the symptoms. Soothing creams and gels with a menthol or alcohol base will in some cases give temporary symptomatic relief. The nail professional should recommend skin products that are soothing to clients with this condition. If the complaint is severe or if you have any question of an underlying disease process, refer the client to a physician for an evaluation.

Neuroma (Neurofibroma, Morton's Neuroma)

In 1876, T. G. Morton described a painful condition in the fourth toe experienced by patients while walking and wearing shoes. In a second paper written in 1886 he stated that he had seen instances of this condition in the third toe also. The pain described with this condition was one of intense spasms or cramping in the forefoot accompanied on occasion with a tingling or electric shock-like feeling into the toes. There may also be a partial loss of feeling in the affected toes. Morton originally attributed this condition to improperly fitting shoes.

What Morton was actually describing is a condition we now know to be a **neuroma** or more precisely a **neurofibroma** of one of the plantar intermetatarsal nerves (Figure 4-21). It is much easier to think of this problem as a scar formation around the nerve where it divides before going into the toes. This scar is generally formed as the result of multiple small injuries to the nerve over a long period of time. The abnormal biomechanics caused in the pronated foot in most instances is the causative factor for this condition. Shoes may be an aggravating factor but there is no real corollary between the type of shoes and the symptoms related to neuroma. The condition may be present in any area where there is a chronic irritation to a nerve, not only between the third and fourth toe.

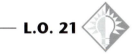
L.O. 21

During the early formation of a neurofibroma clients may experience occasional tingling or electric shock-like feelings in the toes when they are walking. As the condition becomes more severe the symptoms progress to cramping and sharp stabbing or burning pains. These pains will cause the individual to stop walking and at times even to remove shoes to relieve the pain. Early treatment consists of educating the individual about what the problem is and what causes it. Injections of cortisone will sometimes give temporary relief. When the individual no longer wishes to tolerate the pain, a surgical removal of the scarred portion of the nerve is the treatment of choice. This will result in a partial, permanent numbness of the affected toes. This numbness will not cause a problem with balance or walking.

As a nail professional you will have clients with this condition. They will probably tell you they have arthritis in their toes or attribute the pain to their shoes or a callus that may be present in the area of their discomfort. The severity and type of pain is the clue that should alert you to the fact

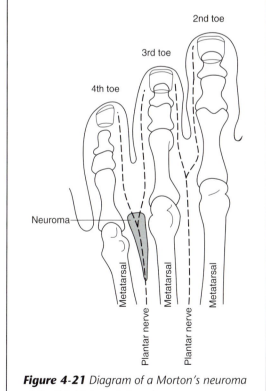

Figure 4-21 *Diagram of a Morton's neuroma of the third intermetatarsal space*

that a neurofibroma may be the cause of their discomfort. Nothing hurts like nerve pain! Clients will not tell you that the nerve hurts because they do not know what is actually causing the problem. They will attribute the symptoms to something they do understand such as arthritis or a callus. By being able to recognize this condition and discussing its possible causes with your clients you will be doing them a great service. Refer them to a podiatrist for a more in-depth workup and treatment.

Heel Pain

For some reason this has become one of the most common complaints in podiatry. Twenty years ago it was much less common. In those years we would take an x-ray of the heel. If a bone spur was present on the bottom of the heel we would tell the patient that to cure the painful heel we needed to surgically remove the spur. The problem was that at least 50% of these patients did not get relief from their complaint. This was an unacceptable cure rate. Over the years we have found the more conservative approach to treatment gives about a 93% cure rate. The other 7% who will need surgery have over a 90% chance of a cure. Why we are seeing so many more heel pain complaints now than we did before remains somewhat of a mystery.

L.O. 22 —— There does not seem to be one common denominator that all heel pain patients share. The complaint is in all age groups, overweight and skinny individuals, those who work on cement surfaces as well as those who have desk jobs. A heel spur may or may not be associated with the condition. Even if there is a spur it in itself is not the cause of the pain. Improper biomechanics resulting in an extra stretch on the plantar fascia where it inserts into the calcaneous seems to be the biggest aggravating factor causing this condition. The majority of the people who have heel pain have an abnormally pronated foot and by using an orthotic to control the pronation, the condition will resolve. On occasion a cortisone shot is needed for those who are in the acute stages of the problem.

Your clients who have this problem will tell you that the first few steps in the morning and after sitting are acutely painful. The reason for this is the plantar fascia is stretched and inflamed where it inserts into the heel bone (Figure 4-22). Inflammation causes swelling and under non-weight-bearing conditions the inflamed area will swell more than when the client is walking on it. Being more swollen and hard after non-weight-bearing movement actually causes more pressure in the area as the

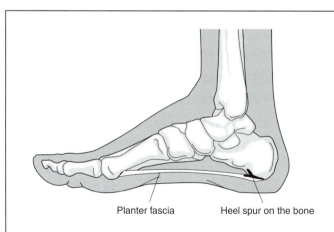

Planter fascia   Heel spur on the bone

Figure 4-22 *This diagram shows how the plantar fascia inserts into the heel bone (calcaneous). If a heel spur is present it is invested in the plantar fascia and it is parallel with the bottom of the foot.*

client begins to walk. This in turn causes more pain. The pressure of the first few steps is actually squeezing the extra swelling out of the heel thus reducing the pressure on the nerve endings. You should advise these clients to wear supportive athletic style walking shoes whenever they are walking. These shoes should be worn even in the evenings around the house; otherwise what is gained during the day is lost in the evening. In some individuals this will reverse the process and make them comfortable. Clients who do not get better should be referred to a podiatrist for a workup and medical treatment for the condition.

FOOT NOTES

At the beginning of this chapter we noted that it should be used for a reference for common foot problems. We hope you will do so and because of it your clients will be better served. Remember many things you will see on or within the foot are the result of abnormal foot function. If you never forget this one fact you will be well equipped to observe the foot in a more critical manner. If you see something on a client that is not discussed here ask your local podiatrist about it.

QUESTIONS

1. When does the adaptive phase of gait start? When does it end?
2. What is the difference between an orthotic and an arch support?
3. What are the three innovations in shoe construction from the 19th century that revolutionized the shoe industry?
4. What is the difference in length between one shoe size and the next?
5. What is a shoe last?
6. What is the "Golden Rule" as it relates to the feet?
7. Why does the skin form a callus?
8. What is the difference between a corn and a callus?
9. What is the difference between a wart and a callus when seen on the bottom of the foot?
10. What are the three most common bacteria found on the surface of our body?
11. What are the only skin glands found on the sole of the foot?
12. What is a common cause of cold feet?
13. What is a Morton's neuroma and what are its symptoms?

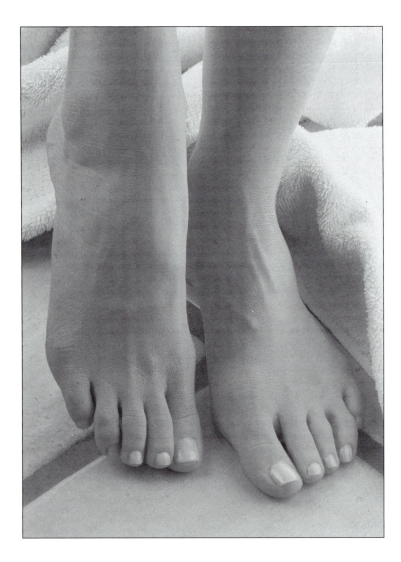

Toenails 5

After studying this chapter, the reader should be able to:

1. Describe the six basic parts of the normal nail module and their functions.

2. Describe the process of nail growth.

3. List the factors that determine the shape of a normal nail.

4. Describe the chemical content of a normal nail.

5. List the four classifications of nail plate problem areas and types of disorders.

6. Describe the process of determining the type of nail disorder.

7. Define the terms pertaining to the nails.

8. Describe five surface irregularities of the nail plate.

9. Describe three main malformations of the nail pate.

10. Describe seven types of soft tissue disorders of the nail plate.

11. Describe a fungal infection in the nail, including the causes, process, and treatment.

12. Describe ten common disorders that affect the tissues surrounding the nail plate.

13. Outline the significance of various changes in nail color.

Toenails for some reason have developed a mystique of their own over the ages. Many "old wives' tales" concerning proper care of the toenails have been around so long that they are today taken as absolute truths. "To prevent ingrown toenails one must cut the nail straight across." "Cut a V in the center of the free edge of the nail to prevent an ingrown nail." To deviate from the practices that they expound will bring nothing but dire consequences to the health of toenails! How many people live with the guilt of not following these rules. "If only I had listened to mom and not cut my nail round I would not now have to suffer with this painful nail." This chapter will help to dispel some of these myths and give you a better understanding of the toenail and some of the common problems related to it.

To understand nail disorders, toenails or fingernails, it is necessary to understand what constitutes a normal nail. The initial discussion in this chapter goes into some depth on the subject of the normal nail. By understanding how the nail plate is formed and grows from the matrix bed to its free edge you will be better able to understand why particular nail disorders occur. Fingernails and toenails have the same basic elements that form the nail plate. They are shaped differently and the reasons for this are discussed. Because we walk on our feet the forces exerted through the toes and thus the toenails are tremendous. These forces magnify any disorders of the toenails as compared to a similar disorder in the fingernails. Footgear adds extra stress and creates a warm, moist environment that complicates as well as creates many nail disorders one does not see in the hands. When looking at the toenails of a client always keep these facts in mind when trying to decide what may be causing or contributing to a nail disorder.

Dismiss the "old wives' tales." They are WRONG and will only get you into trouble!

THE NORMAL NAIL

The normal nail has several different functions. In humans and primates it is adapted to enhance the use of the fingers for handling small objects. It is also used for scratching and grooming purposes as well as having a protective function for the tips of the fingers and toes. In humans alone nails also are used to produce esthetic as well as cosmetic functions. We are well aware of the many manipulations and modifications that may be applied to the nails to enhance their beauty or appearance.

It is important to remember that the nail plate is only the visible structure of a complex group of microscopic structures (the nail module) that actually produce the plate. Too many times when a deformity or abnormality of the plate is observed we fail to look to those deeper structures for answers as to why the particular problem is present. By treating the visible abnormality it is mistakenly thought that the condition will be corrected. As a nail professional you must always understand this and look under the surface of the nail plate for the source of the abnormal condition of the nail. The cause or origin of the problem, in most instances, will be easily understood or identified. You will then be better equipped to recommend services, products, or

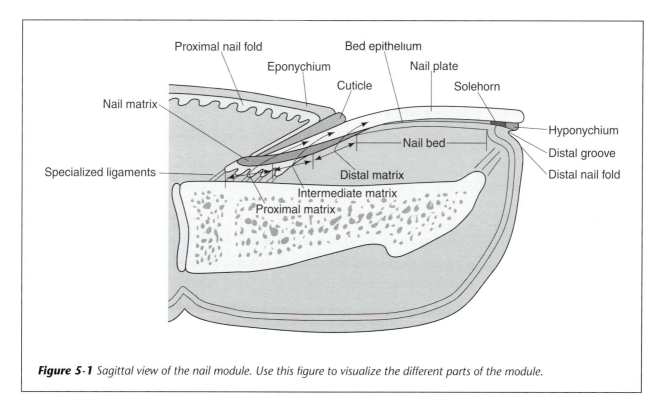

Figure 5-1 *Sagittal view of the nail module. Use this figure to visualize the different parts of the module.*

referrals to other nail specialists that will be of benefit to your client. For these reasons it is imperative for the nail professional to understand the anatomy and growth patterns of the normal nail.

The normal **nail module** (Figure 5-1), as we will call it, is composed of six basic parts: **matrix bed, nail plate, cuticular system (cuticle, eponychium, hyponychium), nail bed, specialized ligaments, and nail folds**.

Matrix Bed. The matrix bed is composed of matrix cells that produce the nail plate. It extends from under the proximal nail groove where it can be seen as a whitish area under the nail plate. This visible portion of the matrix bed is called the **lunula**.

Nail Plate. The nail plate is the most visible and functional part of the nail module.

Cuticular System. The proximal nail fold is the fold of skin at the base or proximal portion of the nail. We see the top of this fold as normal skin. This skin then folds back under itself onto the surface of the nail extending proximally to where the matrix bed begins nail formation. The skin on the under surface of the proximal nail fold adheres to the top of the nail plate and extends out onto the nail as a thin translucent band of the stratum corneum of the epidermal layer of the skin. This is what we see as the **cuticle** or **eponychium**. The true cuticle is under the proximal nail fold extending back to that point where nail is actually being formed at the base of the matrix bed. By its attachment to the nail the true cuticle seals the area against foreign material and microorganisms, thus helping to prevent injury and infection. For this reason the nail professional should not be too aggressive in removing cuticle during a pedicure or manicure service.

The counterpart to the proximal nail fold and eponychium is the **hyponychium** that is found at the distal aspect or free edge of the nail. The hyponychium lies under the nail plate where the free edge of the nail attaches to the underlying tissues. It seals the free edge of the nail to the normal skin thus preventing external moisture, bacteria, or fungi from getting under the nail.

Nail Bed. The nail bed lies under the nail plate and on top of the distal phalanx of the finger or toe. Because it is richly supplied with blood vessels it is observed under the nail plate as a reddish area extending from the lunula to the area just before the free edge of the nail. The nail is attached to the nail bed by a thin layer of tissue called the **bed epithelium**.

At the distal end of the nail bed the bed epithelium meets the hyponychium where it becomes **cornified** and thicker. Here it forms a grayish band that is called the **onychodermal band** or **solehorn** of the nail. The onychodermal band is a combination buildup of bed epithelium and hyponychial tissue. It plays a major role in attaching the nail plate to the underlying tissues. It serves a similar function as does the true cuticle of the proximal nail fold helping to seal the free edge of the nail to the skin. The free edge of the nail plate begins immediately beyond the onychodermal band and hyponychium.

Specialized Ligaments. Specialized ligaments anchor the nail bed and matrix bed to the underlying bone. These ligaments are located at the proximal aspect of the matrix bed and around the edges of the nail bed approximately corresponding to the areas under the nail grooves.

Nail Folds. Nail folds are folds of normal skin that surround the nail plate. These folds of skin form the nail grooves and also serve a minor role in determining the shape of the nail.

Nail Growth

The normal growth rate of fingernails is 0.1 mm per day or approximately 3 mm per month. Toenails grow at about half to one-third that rate. To completely replace a fingernail takes about 6 months; to replace a toenail takes 12 to 18 months. The growth rate of nails varies with age, sex, disease states, and temperature. Between ages 10 to 14 the growth rate peaks and gradually decreases with the aging process. Men's nails generally grow faster than women's. Certain diseases such as psoriasis cause the growth rate to increase. Other disease states such as arteriosclerosis, severe infections, high fevers, and paralysis or inactivity all decrease the growth rate of the nail. Cold tempera-

Fingernails grow somewhat more rapidly than toenails with the rate of growth dependent on many factors.

tures decrease the growth rate; warm temperatures increase it. These are generalities and there are variations between individuals. In general, under normal conditions members of the same family will have similar growth rates of their nails indicating that we may inherit a factor that determines how fast our nails will grow.

The nail plate originates from the matrix bed. The shape and thickness of the nail is determined by the shape of the matrix bed as well as how fast it produces nail plate. The matrix bed may be roughly divided into three areas. These are the proximal matrix, the intermediate or middle matrix bed, and the distal matrix bed. The nail plate grows from the proximal matrix, the central area of the matrix, as well as from the distal aspect of the matrix. The distal aspect of the matrix is

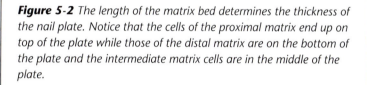
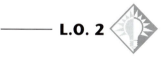

Figure 5-2 *The length of the matrix bed determines the thickness of the nail plate. Notice that the cells of the proximal matrix end up on top of the plate while those of the distal matrix are on the bottom of the plate and the intermediate matrix cells are in the middle of the plate.*

generally seen as that area where the lunula stops and nail bed begins. The length of the matrix bed (Figure 5-2) in an individual will determine the normal nail thickness (approximately 0.5 mm in women and 0.6 mm in men). This is because more matrix will be formed in a longer matrix bed making a thicker nail plate than a nail that would be produced by a short matrix bed.

L.O. 2

The cells at the base of the matrix bed form the top of the plate; those produced at the distal end of the matrix bed form the bottom of the plate. The nail plate therefore is a multilayered structure. The matrix cells at the base of the matrix bed form nail plate faster than those at the distal part of the bed. The underlying or deep layers of the nail plate move forward on the nail bed at a slower rate than do the surface layers of the nail. As long as the rate of nail plate production remains constant the nail will have a "normal" thickness. When abnormal conditions in the matrix occur because of infections, disease, or injury the shape or thickness of the nail plate will change.

The nail plate is attached to the nail bed by a layer of tissue called the bed epithelium. The bed epithelium originates from the distal aspect of the matrix bed. By attaching the nail plate to the nail bed it forces the plate to grow toward the end of the digit instead of growing straight up off the matrix bed. The bed epithelium is tightly attached to the nail plate and loosely

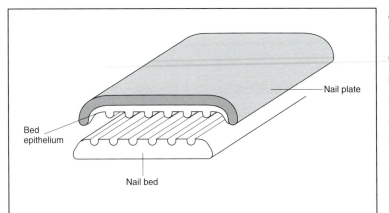

Bed epithelium

Nail plate

Nail bed

Figure 5-3 *The bed epithelium is tightly attached to the nail plate. Notice the grooves in the nail bed which correspond to the ridges in the bed epithelium.*

attached to the nail bed. The top of the nail bed has microscopic grooves in it extending from the distal matrix bed (lunula) to the solehorn or onychodermal band. The bed epithelium has ridges that correspond to the grooves in the nail bed (Figure 5-3). As the nail plate grows the bed epithelium glides over the nail bed rather than the nail moving over the bed epithelium. The grooves and ridges keep the nail plate growing along a straight path from the matrix bed to its free edge. They also make a larger surface area for the bed epithelium to attach to the nail bed.

Where the nail plate passes over the onychodermal band the free edge begins. Remnants of the bed epithelium and the onychodermal band remain attached to the undersurface of the nail as a cuticle or part of the hyponychium. The shape of the nail at this point generally corresponds to the arc shape of the lunula. From this point on the shape of the free edge is determined by environmental factors and personal preferences.

Shape of the Nail

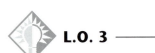

L.O. 3

The shape of the normal nail is determined by a number of different factors:

- Width and length of the matrix bed

- Length of the nail bed

- Shape of the underlying bone

- Environmental factors

- Personal preferences

The matrix bed forms the nail plate we see.

The various combinations of these factors account for the differences we see in the shapes of fingernails as compared to toenails.

The shape of the matrix bed, as a general statement, is the major factor in determining the shape of the nail plate. This is because the matrix bed cells are the only cells that actually contribute to the formation of the nail plate. Other factors help to influence the shape of the matrix bed, but it is still the matrix bed that forms the nail plate we see. If the matrix bed is arched the nail will have an arched shape. If the matrix bed is wide and flat the nail will be wide and flat. If the length of the matrix bed is short then the nail will be thin, and conversely, if the bed is long the nail plate will be thick because more matrix cells are added to the plate as it is formed.

The length of the nail bed is generally longer in fingers than in toes because the distal phalanx in fingers is longer than that in the toes. The extra length of underlying bone provides more attachment for a longer nail bed, which, in turn, results in the longer nail plate seen in the fingers (Figure 5-4). The cross section of the nail plate in fingernails is generally flatter, whereas toenails have a more arched or C-shaped appearance. The shape of the underlying phalanx is the cause. The top of the distal phalanx in the fingers is flat as compared to the convex shape of the distal phalanx in the toes. Because the matrix bed and nail bed are attached to the underlying bone, their shape is more convex in the toe than in the finger. The difference in the longitudinal shape of the nail is also a result of the difference in the shapes of the distal phalanges of fingers and toes. The short stubby distal phalanges of the toes have a downward curve at the end resulting in the nail plate curving down over the end of the toe as compared to the more flat horizontal finger nail plate (Figure 5-5).

The environmental factors that affect the nail shape are mainly the types of jobs different individuals do. Manual laborers, cement masons, and mechanics all work with their hands. As a result of this the nails are worn off short and become thin and may even lose their normal appearance. Cosmetic shapes are a preference of the individual as we are well aware.

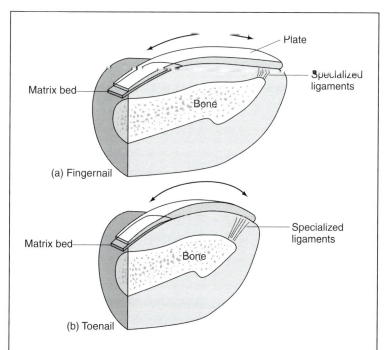

Figure 5-4 The length of the underlying bone helps to determine the length of the nail plate. The distal phalanx of the toe angles down thus the toenail curves down at the free edge because of the attachment of the specialized ligaments.

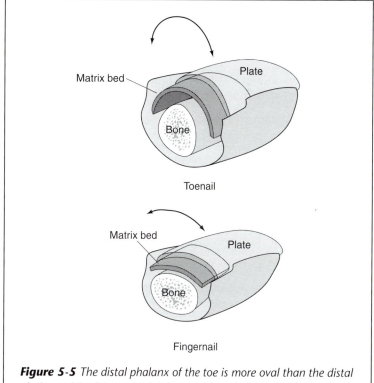

Figure 5-5 The distal phalanx of the toe is more oval than the distal phalanx of the finger which is flatter. This produces a nail plate with a greater side-to-side C shape because the matrix bed is more curved on the sides since it is attached to the underlying bone by the specialized ligaments.

Chemical Content of the Nail

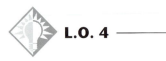

L.O. 4

What is the normal nail plate actually composed of? This is a much studied topic with little universal agreement. Scientific literature seems to agree that the calcium content of nails is overrated. It is present but does not function to make the nail plate stronger or harder. In all probability its presence is not necessary for a healthy nail plate. Other **inorganic** elements also found in the nail plate include magnesium, sodium, potassium, iron, copper, zinc, sulfur, and nitrogen. Sulfur and nitrogen are usually found as chemical parts of **organic** compounds (amino acids) found in the nail. Sulfur is found almost exclusively in the amino acid cystine. Other amino acids are also present and combine to form the main compounds of the nail plate that are, like hair and epidermis, fibrous proteins called keratins.

Nails are not large, but they contain many elements!

The nail is porous and water will pass through it much more easily than through normal skin. The water content of the nail is related to the relative humidity of the surrounding environment. Although they seem to be a dry hard plate, nails have between 10% and 30% water content. The water content of the nail is directly related to its flexibility. The lower the water content in the nail the more brittle it becomes. The application of nail enamel or an ointment-based nail conditioner on the nail plate will reduce the loss of water from the nail.

FOOT NOTES

It is important to understand how a normal nail plate is formed to properly evaluate and identify a nail disorder. By knowing the function of each individual structure that makes up a normal nail module you will generally be able to determine the cause and location of the disorder that is affecting the nail plate. Remember the plate is all you actually see. You need to look under the plate to determine why you are seeing what you see!

DETERMINING LOCATION OF DISORDERS OF THE NAIL PLATE

L.O. 5

Nail plate disorders can be roughly classified into four individual problem areas:

1. Problems that affect the matrix bed

2. Problems that affect the nail bed and bed epithelium

3. Problems that affect the eponychium and hyponychium

4. Problems that affect the structures surrounding the nail plate such as the nail folds or the underlying bone

The previous section discussed how each of these parts of the nail module are related to the nail plate itself. The appearance of the nail plate can give us an idea about which structures within the nail module are causing the particular disorder.

——— **L.O. 5**

◆ Matrix bed problems are generally associated with nail thickness as well as some surface irregularities of the plate. The proximal matrix bed cells form the surface of the nail plate, the middle portion of the matrix bed forms the middle layers of the nail, and the distal portion of the matrix forms the bottom layers of the nail plate. If a disorder of the plate is on the surface it can be generally determined that there is a problem in the proximal matrix bed. If the plate is thick then the disorder is affecting the whole matrix bed. This is also true for thin nails. Grooves or ridges across the nails are rate of growth disturbances within the entire matrix bed.

◆ Nail bed disorders generally are the cause of the nail being loose (detached) from the underlying tissue (**onycholysis**). A buildup of debris and callus under the plate is also generally a nail bed problem. Distortional or misalignment abnormalities of the nail plate in most instances can be traced to bed epithelium injuries or disorders. Bed epithelial problems may also cause onycholysis.

A buildup of debris and callus under the plate is generally a nail bed problem.

◆ Eponychial and hyponychial disorders are associated with **pterygium** (abnormal adherence of the skin to the nail plate) formation. Some surface disorders on the nail plate or under the free edge are also associated with eponychial and hyponychial problems.

◆ Injuries or chronic infections of the nail folds may affect the shape and texture of the nail plate. Problems affecting the shape of the underlying bone will also affect the shape of the nail plate.

The nails of 10% to 50% of patients with psoriasis are affected by the disease. The following is a discussion of psoriasis of the nail module. This particular disease process may affect one or all of the structures within the nail module. This discussion demonstrates how to look at a particular disorder of the nail, psoriasis, and determine why the nail plate appears as it does. Any nail disorder should be looked at in a similar manner to determine a probable cause of that particular disorder.

♦ If the proximal matrix bed is involved, pitting on the surface of the nail will be observed. Transverse grooves across the nail may be observed. These are caused as the disease process intermittently gets better or worse.

♦ Intermediate matrix bed involvement will cause white lines or spots to occur within the nail.

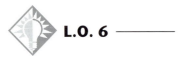

L.O. 6 ———

♦ Distal matrix involvement will cause some thinning of the nail. Small nonadherent areas of nail to the nail bed as the nail grows out may also appear. These are actually "pits" in reverse because the distal matrix forms the under surface of the nail. If the entire matrix bed is involved the nail plate is not formed and if any is formed it will be **dystrophic**, soft, and crumbly.

♦ When the nail bed is involved large amounts of hyperkeratotic tissue are laid down under the nail plate, lifting it up off the bed. This will cause an apparent thickening of the nail. The plate may also come loose from the underlying bed. If the disease is not severe the bed may appear to have reddish brown spots within it. This is the so-called oil drop sign. There may also be small bleeding areas under the nail that appear as **splinter hemorrhages** (discussed later). Because of their close association hyponychial psoriatic nail plate changes resemble those seen in nail bed disease. If the hyponychium detaches from the nail plate, secondary infections from fungus and bacteria may begin affecting the nail module.

Psoriasis can have many effects on the nails of those with the disease.

♦ Psoriasis of the nail folds or grooves will affect the nail plate by causing changes in the growth pattern. Nail grooving and other changes like those already discussed will occur depending on the severity of the disease in these areas. Psoriatic arthritis causes bone destruction of portions of the distal and intermediate phalanges. If the distal phalanx or interphalangeal joint is affected, the nail may become malformed because of the malformation of the underlying bone.

This discussion of the psoriatic nail demonstrates how each anatomic structure of the nail module affects the nail plate. More importantly, it demonstrates how to evaluate any nail plate when trying to determine what is causing the visible changes observed in the nails of your clients.

TOENAIL DISORDERS

With a better understanding of how a normal nail plate is formed and affected by the various parts of the nail module it will be easier to understand the more common toenail disorders. It is difficult to separate toenails and fingernails in this discussion. The same problems that affect toenails may also be seen in fingernails. The main thing to remember is that our feet are most always covered with shoes and socks, creating an entirely different environment. Compare the feet to a tropical environment where the conditions are most always warm and moist, whereas the hands would be compared to a desert or a more temperate environment. We all know that in the tropics the animals are bigger and there are more and larger bugs and other life forms than are found in the desert. In a sense the same holds true for the toenails. Their problems are exaggerated when compared to the fingernails. More fungal problems are noted. Toenails seem to be more susceptible to infections and injuries. Walking, because of the tremendous pressures applied to the toes, also exaggerates many of the disorders associated with the toenails.

Problems with the toenails and feet are magnified because of the enormous stresses placed on the feet by walking.

Most disorders are caused by many different numbers or combinations of individual problems. The nail plate can be viewed as a series of "mirrors" that give us an insight on the general health and well-being of the individual. Seldom is a single problem associated with a single nail disorder. Nail professionals must be able to recognize that a problem exists and possess a general knowledge about the problem. Then they may talk to the client about the condition and thus be able to provide or not provide a nail service appropriately. You need not be concerned with making a definite medical diagnosis of a nail disorder. If this is necessary, the client should be referred to the appropriate medical specialist such as the podiatrist, dermatologist, or primary care physician for a thorough medical workup.

General Terms

The following are some general nonspecific terms referring to the nail, found in the dictionary (Miller & Keane, 1987):

———— **L.O. 7**

- Onych(o)—word element referring to the nails

- Onychalgia (on"i-kal'je-ah)—pain in the nails

- Onychitis (on"i-ki'tis)—inflammation of the matrix of the nail

- Onychodystrophy (on"i-ko-dis'tro-fe)—malformation of the nail

- Onychoheterotopia (on"i-ko-het"er-oto'pe-ah)—abnormal location of the nails

- Onychoid (on'i-koid)—resembling a fingernail (toenail)

- Onychopathy (on"i-kop'ah-the)—any disease or deformity of the nail

Knowing the medical terms used in discussing nail disorders helps the nail professional.

- Onychosis (on"i-ko'sis)—onychopathy

- Onychotomy (on"i-kot"o-me)—incision or cutting into a nail

- Periungual (per"e-ung'gwal)—the tissues or area around the nail plate

- Subungual (sub-ung'gwal)—the tissues or area under the nail plate

- Ungual (ung'gwal)—pertaining to the nails

These terms are general but must be understood to be able to understand and read other more scientific materials on nails. What follows is a discussion about toenail *onychopathy*.

Surface Irregularities of the Nail Plate

L.O. 8

Longitudinal Lines or Grooves. Extending from the hyponychium to the free edge of the nail plate, these may be caused from inherited traits, injuries to the matrix bed, circulatory disorders, or other disease states. Tumors or cysts within the soft tissues causing pressure on the matrix bed and the normal aging process are also causes. By close observation of the nail plates the nail professional will, in most instances, be able to determine in a general sense the cause of the line or groove.

In most instances these lines or grooves do not cause problems. When splitting of the nail plate occurs along these deformities, the nail will catch on things and cause irritations. If all nails are involved, the cause is probably inherited or from a systemic disease process. If only a few individual nails are involved the cause is likely more localized to those particular nails. If the nail plate is grooved or ridged because of a tumor (i.e., wart or cyst), removal of the tumor will return the plate to its normal appearance.

Onychorrhexis (on"i-ko'rek-sis). Onychorrhexis is a series of narrow parallel grooves extending from the base of the nail plate to its free edge (Figure 5-6). Splitting is common in these grooves. This disorder is seen in diseases of the nail such as lichen planus and psoriasis. It may also be caused by occupational trauma.

Transverse (Beau's) Lines. Beau's lines are actually grooves (not the ridges) that extend from one side of the nail to the other (Figure 5-7). They are caused by the matrix bed either temporarily ceasing to produce nail plate or slowing down the production of the plate. When nail plate production by the matrix bed returns to normal, the groove is the result. By measuring the width of the groove one can determine the duration of the illness that caused the decrease in plate production.

The most common cause of this disorder is systemic disease. High fevers, generalized injuries such as seen in auto accidents, and major surgical procedures will all cause this condition. In some women the menstrual cycle will result in multiple Beau's line formations. These causes generally will affect all 20 nail plates. Localized injury to a nail can result in a Beau's line formation in that individual nail. This condition is sometimes observed after ingrown nail surgery. Chronic infections in the area of the proximal nail fold may also be the cause of this nail plate deformity. Overzealous pedicures or manicures resulting in injury to the eponychium when pushing back or removing the cuticle may also cause Beau's lines.

Explain this condition to your patients by telling them that in the face of severe disease or injury the body will put all of its energy into repairing or healing. The formation of nail plate is not necessary for survival so the energy needed to produce nails is more efficiently used to repair or heal other parts of the body. When this process is complete then the body will again start to produce nails. The resultant grooves seen in the nails are merely indications that the body functioned properly in a trying situation.

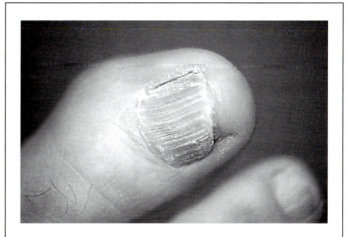

Figure 5-6 Onychorrhexis. Notice grooves in the nail. All of the patient's toenails had these grooves. Possibly this was an inherited problem as no localized or general disease processes were present.

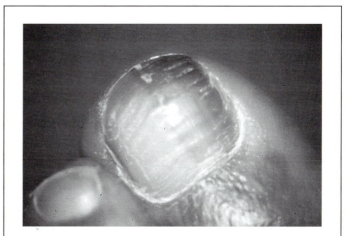

Figure 5-7 Multiple Beau's lines caused by chronic eczema. Notice also the pitting in the nail plate, the result of the eczema affecting the proximal matrix bed as the pits are on the surface of the plate.

Pitting of the Nail Plate. Pitting as seen on the surface of the nail is the result of proximal matrix bed disorders. The most common cause of this disorder in toenails is probably psoriasis. Small traumatic nonpermanent injuries to the matrix may also result in individual pits seen on the plate. Some forms of eczema in the areas of the nail can also cause pitting.

Onychoschizia (on"i-ko'skiz"i-a). Onychoschizia is **lamellar** splitting of the nail plate or splitting of the nail in layers. The area of the nail that is splitting will give a hint as to the cause of this disorder. If the top layer of nail begins to split off in the area of the proximal nail plate then the condition is a systemic disorder such as psoriasis or other disease that affects the proximal matrix bed. Excessive or large doses of vitamin A may also cause onychoschizia.

Distal splitting of the free edge of the nail is generally attributed to repeated exposure to water or certain chemicals. These agents cause hydration and dehydration that results in the separation of the individual layers of the nail plate. Avoidance of these substances will usually result in a cure. The aging process may also produce distal splitting of the plate. As yet no cure for aging has been reported!

Malformations of the Nail Plate

L.O. 9

We have already discussed what the normal nail plate should look like. This section names and discusses abnormal **configurations** or **malformations** of the plate.

Clubbing of the Nail Plate. Clubbing refers to a deformity of the plate that causes excessive curvature from front to back and from side to side. There is also enlargement of the soft tissue structures on the tips of the fingers and toes. The cause of clubbing in 80% of the cases is a decrease of the oxygen in the red blood cells (**hypoxia**). In some instances the nail bed may appear blue (cyanotic) because of the decrease in oxygen to this area. Causes of hypoxia include emphysema, chronic lung infections, chronic heart disease, chronic blood loss, and others. In rare instances single digits may be involved as the result of localized injuries to the blood supply. Chronic infections of the digit may also cause a reduction in the blood supply to the end of the digit that will result in clubbing. This condition is seen mainly in fingernails but if the cause is chronic all 20 nails will be clubbed.

Hypoxia is the cause of 80% of the cases of nail clubbing.

Koilonychia. Koilonychia refers to spoon-shaped nails (Figure 5-8). It is the opposite of clubbing of the nail in that the free edges of the nail turn up, causing the distinctive spoon shape. The tissues under these nails may be normal or have a hyperkeratotic buildup in the sole horn or hyponychial band area. Psoriasis should be ruled out as a cause if there is a thickening in hyponychial band area. The most common causes of this disorder are occupational softening of the nail plate and chronic iron deficiency anemias. Conditions such as arteriosclerosis and aging, which result in thinning of the nail plate, may also result in this disorder. Babies shortly after birth normally exhibit this nail deformity but within a number of months the nail plate will appear normal.

Transverse Nail Deformities. This deformity of the plate (overcurvature of the nail from side to side) is divided into three categories: the pincer or trumpet deformity, the tile

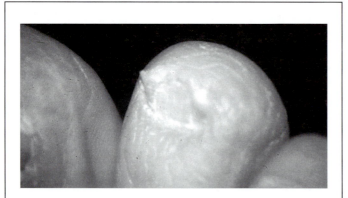

Figure 5-8 *Koilonychia. The plate is adherent to the nail bed but curls up around the free edges.*

shape, and plicatured nail. All three shapes are easily identified in the toenails. The plicatured and pincer or trumpet deformities seem to be more common in the toenails than in the fingernails.

◆ **Trumpet or pincer nail** deformities begin as a normal nail configuration in the matrix area. As the nail grows toward the end of the digit the edges of the plate begin to curl inward. When the nail reaches the end of the digit, depending on the severity of the deformity, it may curl completely in on itself and appear as a trumpet or cone formation (Figure 5-9). The underlying nail bed and distal skin are constricted within this curl and may become painful. Causes of this deformity may be a bone spur on the top of the underlying bone. However, the most likely cause is an inherited disorder. On very rare occasions improperly fit shoes may produce the deformity.

◆ **Tile-shaped nails** have an increased transverse curvature throughout the nail plate (Figure 5-10). The curve is caused by an increased curvature of the matrix bed. The borders of the nail are parallel with each other. This nail type will not cause discomfort to the individual.

◆ **Plicatured** (plik'a-choor'ed) **nail** deformity figuratively means folded nail (Figure 5-11). The surface of the nail is generally flat while one or both of the edges of the plate are folded at a 90° or more angle down into the soft tissue margins. This deformity originates at the matrix bed. The bed is folded causing the plate to be formed in the plicatured fashion. This nail deformity is most often seen as the cause of ingrown nails in the toes. This disorder may result from an injury that deforms the matrix bed. Shoe pressure over a period of time may result in a remolding and folding of the matrix bed in this manner. This deformity may also be inherited.

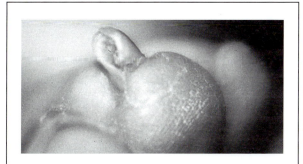

Figure 5-9 Trumpet nail of the second toe; may be the result of chronic injury as the toe is longer than the others.

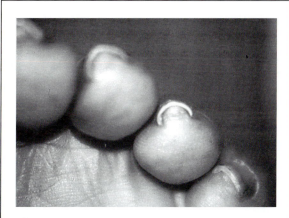

Figure 5-10 The third and fourth toenails on this foot demonstrate a tile shape.

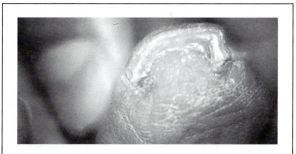

Figure 5-11 A Plicatured nail deformity. This nail was sanded down to better show the right angle fold on the nail margin. Also notice the thickening of the solehorn as the result of a chronic fungal infection of the nail bed.

L.O. 10 ———— **Pterygium (Ta-rij'e-am).** This term is defined in the medical dictionary as a wing-like structure. It relates to the nail when the eponychium or hyponychium abnormally adheres to the nail plate. Dorsal pterygium occurs on the top of the plate when the eponychium and true cuticle abnormally attach to the nail plate (Figure 5-12). As the nail grows the proximal nail fold is stretched over the nail forming the wing-like extension of skin. In severe cases the cuticle may adhere to the matrix stopping plate formation in that area, which results in a split in the nail. If the process continues the entire matrix bed may become adherent to the cuticle causing the loss of the nail plate (Figure 5-13).

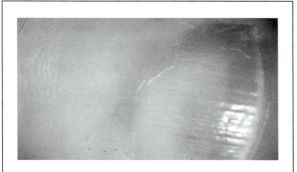

Figure 5-12 Pterygium formation on the top of the nail showing a wing-like process of skin abnormally adhered to the nail plate. This is probably the result of an injury.

The opposite of dorsal pterygium is ventral pterygium. This process involves the free edge of the nail with the hyponychium remaining adherent to the underlying portion of the plate. In this disorder the distal nail groove is eliminated. The hyponychium will appear thickened because of this.

The most common cause of dorsal pterygium is lichen planus. Ventral pterygium is most often associated with Raynaud's disease as seen with scleroderma and also arteriosclerosis. Dorsal or ventral pterygium associated with disease processes generally affects more than one nail. Traumatic pterygium formation generally involves only the injured nail. There are also congenital forms of dorsal and ventral pterygium.

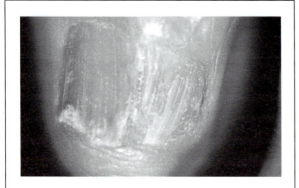

Figure 5-13 Severe pterygium formation has resulted in the loss of nail plate in the area where the skin had adhered to the nail matrix and also the bed. This is the result of rheumatoid arthritis.

Thickening of the Nail Bed and Hyponychium. This disorder is characterized by the formation of hyperkeratotic buildup under the nail plate in the areas of the hyponychium and nail bed. Causes in the toes are generally from improperly fit footgear or a malpositioning of the toes such as hammer or mallet toe deformities. These result in continued minor injuries to the nail module over a long period of time. The underlying tissues thicken as a result of these injuries. Psoriasis, fungal infections (discussed later), and some forms of eczema may also contribute to this condition.

Splinter Hemorrhages. Splinter hemorrhages are the result of bleeding between the nail bed and nail plate (Figure 5-14). They form in the manner they do

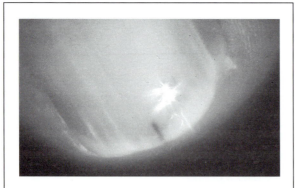

Figure 5-14 This splinter hemorrhage has almost grown out off the nail bed. It appears, as its name implies, like a small splinter under the edge of the nail.

because of the ridges and grooves in the bed epithelium and the top of the nail bed. The blood follows these microchannels, taking on the elongated shape of a "splinter." There are many causes of splinter hemorrhages. Small blood clots associated with bacterial endocarditis usually affect all of the nails. Psoriasis of the nail bed is also a cause and will affect those nails involved in the disease. Rheumatoid arthritis is another common cause also affecting only the involved nails. By far the most common cause are small or microtraumatic injuries to the nail bed.

Subungual Hematoma (he'ma-to'ma). A subungual hematoma or blood clot under the nail plate is different from splinter hemorrhages in that the nail becomes loose from the nail bed, allowing a blood clot to form in the space (Figure 5-15). This is usually the result of traumatic injury to the nail module. A slight traumatic injury to the matrix bed may produce a hemorrhage into the nail plate itself. Remember that the proximal matrix produces the top layers of the plate and the intermediate matrix bed produces the middle layers of the plate, and so on. Therefore, if an injury occurs in the intermediate matrix bed the hematoma will be in the middle layers of the nail plate. Psoriasis in the matrix bed may also cause this disorder. More severe trauma to the nail module will cause the nail plate to lift off the underlying tissues with resultant bleeding in the space produced. This condition may be severely painful, and draining the blood from under the nail will produce instant relief.

Onychomadesis (on"i-ko-mah-de'sis). Onychomadesis or shedding of the nail plate, is characterized by a separation of the nail plate from the matrix bed (Figure 5-16). In most cases the cause can be traced to a localized infection, minor injuries to the matrix bed, or a severe systemic illness. Some chemotherapy treatments or x-ray treatments for cancer may also cause this condition. Localized causes will involve individual nails, but in systemic problems all the nails will usually be involved. This disorder occurs when the matrix bed ceases to produce nail plate for a period of at least one to two weeks. Conditions in which Beau's lines occur are of a shorter length of time so a groove is formed rather than the complete separation of the plate from the matrix as in this disorder. In most cases when the causative factors are removed a new nail plate will form.

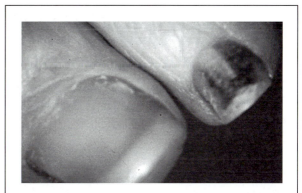

Figure 5-15 *Old injury to the second toenail resulted in bleeding under the nail. At first the color appears a reddish blue but as the blood coagulates it turns brown to black.*

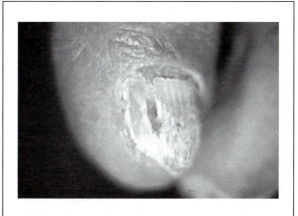

Figure 5-16 *Onychomadesis. This nail is shedding at the matrix bed as a result of a long-standing fungal infection. Notice the new nail pushing the old off as it forms under it.*

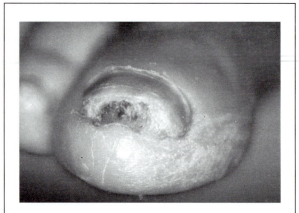

Figure 5-17 *A fungal infection involving the hyponychium. The soft tissues in this area thicken and the nail becomes thick and dystrophic as more of the nail module becomes involved.*

Splinter hemorrhages and subungual hematomas result from traumatic injury to the nail module.

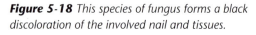 L.O. 11

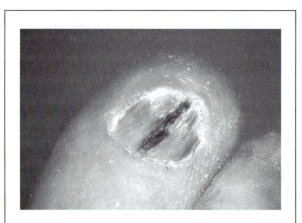

Figure 5-18 *This species of fungus forms a black discoloration of the involved nail and tissues.*

Onycholysis (on"i-kol'i-sis). Onycholysis is a disorder in which the nail plate separates from the nail bed. This nail disorder is basically the opposite of onychomadesis. The plate separates from the free edge back toward the matrix bed. In the foot it is most often associated with bacterial or fungal infections of the nail. Shoe trauma also contributes to this condition. Other causes may include psoriasis of the nail bed, pernicious anemias, and arteriosclerosis.

Onychomycosis (on"i-ko-mi-ko'sis). Onychomycosis, also known as tinea unguium (tin'e-ah un'gium), is the most common disorder of the toenails (Figure 5-17). It is a fungal infection of the nail module. This term also includes yeast infections (candida) of the module. The most common causative organisms associated with this disorder are *Tinea rubrum*, *Tinea mentagrophytes*, and *Candida albicans*. Many other species may also cause this condition. In most instances it is rare that the fungus is the primary problem. Fungi are **saprophytes** which are organisms that live on dead or diseased organic matter. For a fungus to grow these conditions are usually necessary. In most instances a pre-existing localized or systemic disorder is present that lowers the resistance of the nail module.

Fungal infections usually start along the nail margins or under the free edge of the plate. These areas of the toenails remain warm and moist because footgear creates an ideal environment for the growth of fungi. After penetrating the hyponychium the organisms invade the nail bed where they cause thickening and hyperkeratosis of the nail bed and hyponychium. Discoloration and onycholysis of the plate from the bed are later results of the infection. Different colors may be noted (white, yellow, black, green) depending on the species of fungi present (Figure 5-18). Later in the infective process the nail plate becomes involved causing it to break down and take on the crumbly appearance of the typical fungal nail. When the fungus invades the matrix bed the plate becomes misshapen and more crumbly, and the matrix cells may even stop producing nail plate resulting in onychomadesis. Secondary infections by other saprophytes occur in long-standing fungal nail infections.

Fungal infections arising in the nail fold areas and at the free edge of the plate most often are caused by the rubrum and mentagrophytes species of fungus. Proximal nail fold or eponychial fungal infections are not as common because the area tends to remain drier and cleaner than other areas surrounding the nail plate. When they occur the rubrum species is most involved and onychomadesis occurs because of the proximal matrix bed involvement.

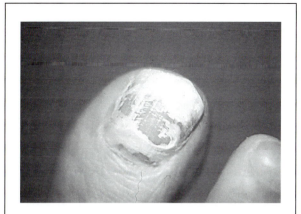

Figure 5-19 *Leukonychia mycotica is a white form of fungus that grows on the surface of the nail plate.*

Fungal infection of the superficial nail plate is a common occurrence in toenails because of the environment created by footgear. This type of fungal infection is most often caused by the mentagrophytes species. It appears as a white discoloration on the surface of the nail. The medical term for this disorder is **leukonychia mycotica** (loo"ko-nik"e-ah mi-kot"i-ca)(Figure 5-19).

Candida or yeast infections of the nail module, as a result of the warm moist environment in which the toenail exists, are relatively common. They usually start in the lateral or proximal nail folds. The soft tissues in these areas become puffy and red. Onycholysis occurs quickly and on removal of the loose portion of nail plate the nail bed is moist and bright red in color as the result of this infection. In some cases where the skin fold is severely involved the superficial layer of skin will slough off also revealing the typical bright red discoloration of the underlying tissue.

Fungal infections of the nails usually occur because of some weakness in the nail module. Fungi are opportunistic in that they take advantage of any weakness of the host organism, in this case the nail and surrounding tissues. Injuries creating a portal of entry for the fungi are taken advantage of. If the individual is debilitated from a disease such as diabetes or arteriosclerosis, the nail module will not be as healthy as it should be and fungi will have an easy time invading it. Prolonged illnesses of any type will have the same affect on the nail modules. Localized disease processes such as psoriasis and or chronic infections of the nail module also allow fungi to begin growing within the nail module. Multiple microinjuries or a single severe injury to the nail module create an unhealthy nail that is less resistant to disease and will allow access for fungi to the area. For these reasons the cuticles on the toenails should not be aggressively reduced when giving a foot service. Any small injuries to the eponychium or hyponychium create portals of entry for fungus to enter the nail module. Placing the foot back into footgear creates the perfect environment for the fungus to infect these injured areas.

Fungal infections of the nails usually occur because of some weakness in the nail module.

Finally, some of us are born with a resistance to fungal infections and others are not. It is unusual to see onychomycosis in children before puberty. After puberty the chances of fungal infections in the nails seems to increase. This suggests an inborn resistance that we lose as we get older. Ask younger infected individuals who have multiple mycotic nails if their parents have the same problem. Their answer usually is that one or both of their parents have severe fungal nail infections. This further substantiates the resistance theory.

Once a fungus has invaded the toenail module the prognosis for curing this disorder is very poor. Numerous treatments have been put forth over the years, all with very little success. If it appears that the entire nail bed and some of the matrix areas are involved a cure is almost impossible. The earlier and less involved the infection, the better the chances are for a resolution of the problem. In most cases of onychomycosis, a primary disease process, localized or generalized, is the predisposing factor. The primary problem must be addressed before any lasting cure for the fungal disorder can be expected.

Fungal infections of the nails are common and opportunistic; treatment is not always successful.

Some practices are having success with the product Clear Nails[®][1]. For the lesser involved toenails it is superior in effectiveness. For more involved toenails it is satisfactory. Like all other topical antifungal nail products it must be used over a long period (many months to well over a year) depending on the severity of the infection. In most instances because of the susceptibility factor it must be used periodically after the disorder is resolved. This is for **prophylaxis** to prevent a recurrence of the infection. If there is a primary cause such as psoriasis, injury to the nail module, or poor circulation, this primary problem must be addressed.

Oral antifungal medications are on the market today. The newer ones are said to be more effective than those we are already using. Griseofulvin has been available for many years. To treat fungal toenails it must be used for many months. In the vast majority of cases the fungus recurs after this medication has been discontinued. New oral medications are being advertised to the public. They work much faster than the older Griseofulvin. If other non-fungal organisms are involved in the disorder, the oral medications do not destroy them. Finally, if there is a primary disease process that allowed the nail to be susceptible to the fungus in the first place, the oral antifungals will do nothing for that. One of the choices I give my patients, who do not wish to live with mycotic toenails, is a permanent total removal of the nail plate (Figure 5-20). Cosmetic appearance and comfort is much better than putting up with a thick mycotic nail or nails. I even see women put polish on the skin surface so that it appears a nail is still present.

When the nail professional notices a fungal infection of the nail, a referral to a dermatologist is in order. The doctor will advise the patient of the various treatment options available. The patient can then make an informed choice on how they wish to have the fungus treated.

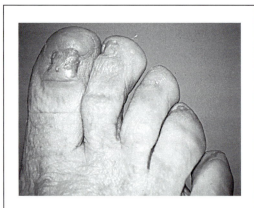

Figure 5-20 *This shows the permanent removal of all the nails. Before this was done the patient was in every 3 months to have the thick painful nails ground down. The final result looks much better than before and the patient can now wear all different styles of shoes with comfort.*

---

[1]Clear Nails[®], Woodward Laboratories Inc., 10357 Los Alamitos Blvd., Los Alamitos, CA 90720.

FOOT NOTES

Onychomycosis or tinea unquium is the most common disorder of the toenails. It is not easily transmitted from one person to another. In the foot it is most commonly caused by *Tinea rubrum* and *Tinea mentagrophytes*, which are fungi, and *Candida albicans*, which is a yeast-like fungi. These are opportunistic organisms that live on dead or diseased organic matter (saprophytes). In most instances the disorder is preceded by a systemic disease process like diabetes or direct injuries to the nail tissues that cause an unhealthy susceptible nail. Because of this the nail professional should not be aggressive in removal of the cuticle during a foot service.

The prognosis for a cure of this disorder is rather poor. If the fungal infection is not severe the better the "cure" rate. Clear Nails® is an acceptable topical medication that can be dispensed by the nail professional. The oral antifungal products are not a satisfactory treatment for onychomycosis of the toenails.

The nail professional should not be apprehensive about giving a pedicure service to a client with onychomycosis. Practicing proper sanitation techniques in the salon (discussed later) will reduce to acceptable levels the possibilities of transferring the fungus to yourself or to other clients. To make a general policy to not give a foot service to individuals with onychomycosis is cutting out a large part of the population from your client base. If you need help with or have a question about a client who has this disorder refer the client to a podiatrist for evaluation before giving the service.

Saprophytes are opportunistic organisms that live on dead or diseased organic matter.

Disorders Affecting the Tissues Surrounding the Nail Plate

Paronychia (par"o-nik'e-ah). Paronychia is an inflammation of the folds of tissue surrounding the nail plate. The organisms that cause this disorder are usually bacteria or fungi. This disorder seems to occur in the toenails more frequently than in fingernails. For this condition to occur there must be a break or weakening of the tissues, portal of entry, to allow the organism entrance to the underlying tissue structures. The warm moist conditions created by footgear is the perfect environment for these organisms to multiply if given the opportunity. Cracking of the skin in the toes is a common occurrence that will contribute to this disorder. The accentuated transverse curvature of toenails associated with the mechanical forces of walking also contributes to injuries of the surrounding soft tissues. Improper trimming of the nails or aggressive manipulation of the cuticle may cause injuries to the tissues resulting in a portal of entry for a pathogenic organism. The nail professional must be aware of these contributing factors when providing a foot service.

L.O. 12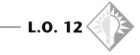

Paronychia may be divided into acute and chronic forms. Acute forms generally occur shortly after there is a break in the skin surrounding the nail plate. Acute forms are most often caused by a bacteria. In the toes this is generally a *Staphylococcus aureus* organism. Candida or yeast organisms may also be involved in the acute form but are more often associated with a chronic paronychia. In acute forms the early stages appear as a localized red swollen area, usually along the nail fold. If allowed to progress, more swelling occurs along with a darker reddish color. The area in the center of the infected site generally will form a small abscess or pus pocket that appears as a whitish yellow color under the skin. Throbbing and acute pain are also present at this stage of the infection. If allowed to continue the infection will involve other areas of the nail module that may result in the loss of the nail plate.

Chronic forms of paronychia are most often the result of candida or fungal organisms invading the soft tissues. They are generally present for some time before being recognized as a problem. Under proper conditions a chronic paronychia may become an acute paronychia. In the chronic form the tissues become inflamed, puffy, and reddened but do not generally form pus pockets or have a drainage. In many instances the disorder is viewed by the individual as an aggravation rather than a potentially serious problem. Psoriasis, diabetes, arteriosclerosis, chronic eczema, and hyperhidrosis are all conditions that may contribute to this disorder. If the chronic form is present for a long period the nail plate will generally show changes in color, shape, or consistency. In long-term chronic cases the nail plate may spontaneously **avulse** from the underlying structures. A new, usually more dystrophic, nail plate will regrow only to repeat the process if the infection is not resolved.

Prevention is the best treatment for paronychia.

The treatment of paronychia depends on the severity of the disorder. Prevention is the best treatment. Proper trimming of the nails and care of the surrounding soft tissues is imperative. The regular use of cuticle creams and moisturizers is recommended. Good foot hygiene is a must. By keeping the tissues surrounding the nail plate as healthy as possible the incidence of paronychia is reduced. If the nail professional accidentally cuts the client when trimming the nail, a disinfectant should be applied. At the end of the service the additional application of a triple antibiotic ointment such as Neosporin®[2] and a small adhesive dressing are recommended. Be sure to advise the client what has happened! People become very dissatisfied with a service if they feel something has been hidden from them. Tell them to keep the area clean and covered for a few days. They should even use the ointment during this time as a precaution against infection. If an acute infection develops or you see a client with an acute infection, the client should be referred

[2]Burroughs Wellcome Co., Research Triangle Park, NC 27709

to the podiatrist for professional medical care. At this point the primary cause of the paronychia must be addressed. Antibiotics may be needed and if an abscess is present it must be drained. Chronic paronychial disorders must be recognized by the nail professional and these clients should also be referred on to the podiatrist for care.

Onychocryptosis (on"i-ko-krip-to'sis). Onychocryptosis or ingrown toenail is discussed here because it is usually seen as an acute paronychia of the soft tissues along the nail margin. This disorder is the result of the matrix bed being folded or involuted deep into the soft tissues. Plicatured nails and tile-shaped nails are most commonly seen associated with this problem. The mechanical forces of walking press the soft tissues up against the nail margin adding to the problem. As the nail grows toward its free edge it encounters a soft tissue wall at the end of the deepened nail groove. At this point it continues growing toward the end of the toe penetrating the soft tissue, thus creating a portal of entry. This results in an acute bacterial paronychia usually caused by *Staphlococcus aureus*. The distal end of the toe becomes red, acutely painful, and a small abscess or pus pocket forms. If the infection persists for any length of time a reddish hamburger-like mass of tissue forms along the edge of the nail. This is called granulation tissue which forms as the result of the body's attempt to heal the infected area (Figure 5-21). Relief from this condition is obtained only by trimming away the offending nail margin and draining the abscess.

The misconceptions about ingrown toenails should be corrected by the nail professional in dealings with clients.

There are many misconceptions and myths concerning this disorder. The first one to dispel is that not trimming the toenails straight across causes ingrown toenails. Anyone who has had an ingrown nail knows the nail cannot be cut straight across and keep it comfortable much less prevent the ingrown nail from occurring! It must be cut back along the margin so that it will not penetrate the soft tissues at the end of the nail groove. The second misconception is that ingrown toenails may be prevented or relieved by cutting a "V" in the end of the nail. The shape of the nail is predetermined by the shape of the matrix bed. A "V" at the distal end of a dead nail plate will not in any way change the shape of that nail plate! A third misconception is that packing cotton under the edge of the nail will help to cure or prevent an ingrown nail. This again attempts to change the shape of an already preshaped nail plate. The only thing the cotton will do is keep the nail from penetrating the skin. If left in place for any length of time the pressure of the nail growing against the cotton packing will begin to cause discomfort and

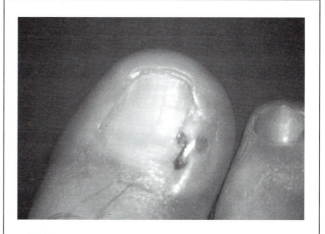

Figure 5-21 *A chronic ingrown nail. Notice the extra granulation tissue that has built up as the result of the nail chronically irritating the tissues.*

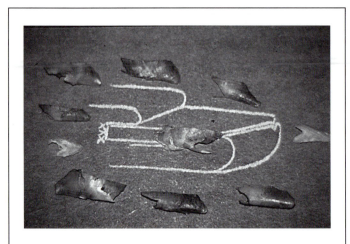

Figure 5-22 *The hook! The diagram shows an actual sidewall of nail that was removed during an ingrown toenail procedure. Notice the large hook that was deeply imbedded in the soft tissue of the nail margin. The others are all sidewalls of nails removed from ingrown nails. They illustrate the various hooks that can be left behind if the nail is improperly trimmed.*

even skin breakdown. As soon as the cotton is removed the ingrown nail will recur because the shape of the nail plate has not been changed. *The nail must be properly trimmed back along the margin to relieve the pressure and prevent the infection that will inevitably occur.*

What does proper trimming of the nail mean? When the border of a toenail is trimmed one has to be very careful not to leave a "hook" or sharp point along the nail edge (Figure 5-22). The trick is not to go too far back along the edge with the nail cutter. If the tip of the nail cutter does not extend slightly beyond the edge of the nail when the cut is made the nail will always break at a 90° angle to the tip of the cutter. This is what causes the so-called hook associated with the ingrown nail. If a hook is left on the edge of the nail, relief from the condition will only last for a short while until the point on the hook grows out to easily penetrate the skin along the margin. These hooks or spicules of nail can penetrate the skin at the end of the toe in severe ingrown nail conditions. A patient may have been trying to "get the hook" but never can trim quite deep enough so the nail keeps breaking off leaving the spicule attached. These toes are extremely swollen and painful and have chronic drainage from the nail margin.

This disorder is easily corrected on a permanent basis in the podiatrist's office. The shape of the matrix bed must be changed. Numerous methods are used to accomplish this. A surgical excision of the folded portion of the matrix bed is one method. With this method there is more pain and disability associated with the procedure than with others. Also the recurrence rate is high because in many cases all the offending matrix fold is not removed because it is hard to visualize. A recommendation may be the simpler phenol technique because there is less pain, disability, and recurrence. With a laser the matrix bed cannot be visualized and therefore not all of the offending matrix cells are destroyed. With the phenol technique the liquid flows into the entire area where the nail plate has been removed destroying all of the matrix cells it comes into contact with. Because the phenol is an acid (carbolic acid) it takes a little longer to heal, but the advantages of this technique outweigh the disadvantages, making it the treatment of choice for many podiatrists.

Calloused Nail Groove. This soft tissue disorder is similar to an ingrown nail with the exception that the discomfort is caused from a callus rather than an infection (Figure 5-23). Again the nail is generally tile shaped

When the border of a toenail is trimmed one has to be very careful not to leave a "hook" or sharp point along the nail edge.

or plicatured. The client will complain of acute pain around the nail whenever there is any pressure on it. The weight of bed sheets is often enough to cause great discomfort. On observation of the nail there will be no soft tissue swelling or heat. There may be slight redness in the soft tissues along the margin but in general it is hard to see any reason for the acute nature of the complaint. There may or may not be visible callus or other debris along the margin. However, when the nail margin is carefully trimmed back a small area of callus will be noted at the distal end of the groove. This is where the nail was pressing into the soft tissue. Most of the time this callus can be easily lifted out of the pocket in which it forms (Figure 5-24). Removal of the nail margin and the callus results in instant relief!

Why this condition occurs rather than the usual infection associated with the ingrown nail is not clear. One explanation may be that the nail is growing extremely slowly allowing the skin time to form the callus to protect itself. The other explanation may be that the individual is not very active so the nail does not get forced through the skin as it does in the more active individual. It seems that this disorder is seen more in the elderly inactive patient than in the younger population. If unable to keep these patients comfortable with proper nail care, recommend a permanent removal of the nail margin by the phenol procedure.

Subungual Keratoma or "Corn." This condition usually presents as a small discolored (yellowish, whitish, or brownish) area under the nail plate. It is a buildup of callus tissue secondary in most instances to improperly fit shoes. The shoe compresses the nail onto the nail bed, which in turn is compressed onto the underlying bone. A callus or "corn" is formed as a result of this pressure. The condition is acutely painful if pressure is applied to the nail plate. This condition may also be associated with a thick nail or a subungual exostosis. Care for this disorder necessitates careful grinding away of the overlying nail plate and trimming of the callus tissue. This is a relatively pain-free procedure and gives immediate relief of discomfort. The nail professional should not attempt to do this for a client; a referral to the podiatrist is necessary.

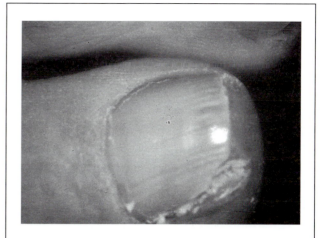

Figure 5-23 *Calloused nail groove. Notice the buildup of callus in the nail groove. The nail has been cut back to relieve the pressure.*

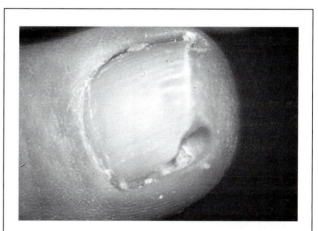

Figure 5-24 *Same toe as in Figure 5-23. The callus has been gently lifted out of the groove to give instant relief from the constant pressure pain associated with this condition. Observe the deep pocket in the groove where the callus has been removed.*

Subungual Exostosis. This is a bony projection extending upward from the distal phalanx causing pressure under the nail plate. Pain on compression of the nail plate is usually the first symptom and as the exostosis enlarges, the plate becomes malformed and more painful. On observation of the plate the underlying nail bed usually has a round whitish area where the exostosis is compressing the blood vessels in the tissues. Applying more pressure causes the white area to increase in diameter and also increases the discomfort. In some instances if the exostosis is projecting up near the free edge of the plate the tissues in this area may have the appearance of a wart. Depending on symptoms the exostosis will need to be surgically removed.

Viral Warts. Warts around or under the nail are not uncommonly associated with toenails. If the wart is large enough to cause pressure on or under the nail plate, a ridge or groove may be formed. These warts are the same as a wart any other place on the body but because of location they cause nail plate disorders. When they are treated the doctor must take care not to injure the underlying nail module, thereby causing permanent damage or malformation of the nail.

Fibromas. Fibromas can occur in the tissues surrounding the nail plate. They appear as smooth pinkish elongated extensions projecting from the skin folds. Depending on size and location they may cause malformation of the nail plate in a manner similar to warts. If they are painful or bothersome they may be removed by the podiatrist.

Fibromas appear as smooth pinkish elongated extensions projecting from the skin folds.

Mucoid Cyst. Some authors say this is an uncommon finding in the toes. This lesion is generally found in the area of the proximal nail fold (Figure 5-25). It generally does not cause pain as long as properly fitted shoes are worn. It appears as a small dome-shaped elevation directly under the skin. As it enlarges the skin becomes thin and has the appearance of a small blister. Because it causes pressure on the matrix bed, a longitudinal groove is formed in the nail. The cyst is attached to the capsule of the underlying joint and is usually filled with a thick clear fluid-like material. Podiatrists have had some success in draining the cyst with a needle and syringe; however, the lesion usually must be surgically excised if the individual desires to get rid of it. Care must be taken not to injure the matrix bed during the removal of the cyst. If injury does occur the future nail plate may be permanently deformed.

Longitudinal Melanonychia (mel"ah-no-nik'e-ah). A longitudinal melanonychia is a black band seen under or within the nail plate extending from the proximal nail fold to the free edge

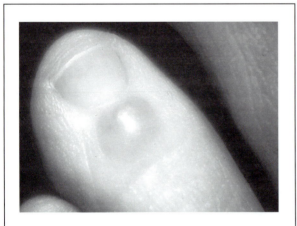

Figure 5-25 *A mucoid cyst at the base of the nail. It is not malignant but as it grows the pressure on the matrix bed can cause a distortion or groove in the nail.*

(Figure 5-26). This condition is caused by a localized area of increased **melanocytes** (pigment cells) usually within the proximal matrix bed. As matrix cells form nail plate, melanin is laid down within the plate by the melanocytes. As the plate grows toward the free edge a dark band of melanin becomes visible. This condition is present in all dark-skinned races. Nearly 100% of blacks over the age of 50 exhibit this condition. This condition is seen in approximately 12% to 25% of the Japanese. In whites it is extremely rare and if seen a malignant melanoma must be suspected and medically ruled out as the cause.

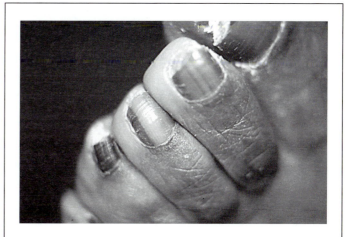

Figure 5-26 All nails on this patient demonstrate melanonychia. The fourth and fifth nails are completely black as a result of melanin deposition in the nail.

Subungual Malignant Melanoma.
This is a serious, potentially life-threatening condition. This malignant lesion of the nail module is found in approximately 2% to 3% of the white population who have a melanoma. In 10% to 15% of the black population who have a melanoma it is exhibited in the nail module. However, because melanomas in general are rare in blacks the actual percentage of the entire black to white population who may have this condition is about equal. The great toe or thumb is most often affected. The condition is usually asymptomatic.

The melanoma may appear as a brown to black spot or band in the matrix bed, nail bed, or the plate itself if it originates in the proximal matrix bed. It may appear as a band or have irregular nondistinct margins. If the discoloration spreads from under the nail into the skin surrounding the nail plate the lesion is almost surely a melanoma. In the dark-skinned races if a longitudinal melanonychial band begins to widen or the edges become less distinct a melanoma must be ruled out. About 25% of the melanomas of the nail module are amelanotic (without melanin) and may appear as a reddish or pink color. In the nail module they will mimic the granulation tissue associated with chronic ingrown nails.

Melanoma may appear as a brown to black spot or band in the matrix bed, nail bed, or the plate itself.

Delayed diagnosis of this serious but rare condition increases the death rate for those individuals who may have it. The nail professional, whose primary focus is working with the nails, may be the first person to suspect the client may have this condition. It is therefore important that any suspicious lesion of the nail module be referred to a medical specialist for a definitive diagnosis. The old adage "It is better to be safe than sorry" must always be followed if there is even a suspicion of this disorder. The earlier the diagnosis is made the greater the chances are for a total cure.

Chromonychia (kro"mo-nik'e-ah)

This section discusses color changes in the nail plate and on its surface (**chromonchia**). Some color changes such as melanonychia and changes seen in fungal infections of the nail module and plate have already been discussed. In many cases it may be hard or impossible to determine the exact cause of the color change. As a general statement Zaias (1980) has postulated that if a discoloration follows the shape of the lunula an internal cause is most likely. When the discoloration follows the shape of the proximal nail fold the cause is more likely from external factors. It is important to look at all 20 nails in trying to determine what may be the most likely causative factor in the color change. If only a few of the nails or a single nail are involved a local cause should be expected. If all 20 are involved a more generalized problem is most likely the causative factor. The way light is refracted through the nail plate will affect the color appearance of the nail. Is the color change in the plate, on top of the plate, or under the plate? It is critical to be observant when trying to determine why a particular color change may be seen in the nail.

Leukonychia (loo"ko-nik'e-ah). Leukonychia, or white nails, is the most common color change seen in the nails. The entire nail may be affected but more usually only portions of the nail show this color change. In some instances the plate may appear whitish because of an underlying disorder of the subungual tissues or a lysis of the plate from the nail bed. Certain species of fungal infections will cause this disorder.

Muehrcke's Bands or Lines. These are a series of transverse white bands separated by pink areas and parallel to the lunula. They are apparent leukonychia in that they are not a discoloration of the nail plate. They are caused by an abnormality of the vascular structures within the nail bed. These lines disappear if the nail plate is compressed on the nail bed. It is theorized they represent localized areas of swelling in the nail bed as the result of increased levels of albumin, a protein, in the liquid portion of the blood (serum albumin). When normal serum albumin levels return the lines disappear. Diseases of the liver or kidneys and malnutrition are disorders that may increase the albumin levels.

Mees' Lines. These are transverse white lines that are actual changes in the nail plate. They do not disappear on compression of the nail plate on the nail bed. They follow the shape of the lunula. They are the result of systemically induced injuries to the matrix bed. Classic Mees' lines are associated with arsenic poisoning. However, acute toxic poisoning from any one of a number of causes may result in this disorder. Mees' lines have little significance because they are an aftereffect of a more acute and usually life-threatening problem.

L.O. 13

Changes in the color of nails are often clues to many systemic diseases or injuries to the nails themselves.

Transverse White Lines. These lines that duplicate the shape of the proximal nail fold are usually from injuries to the nail fold and underlying matrix areas. They may extend entirely across the plate or only partially. Because of the matrix involvement the discoloration is within the plate itself. They are usually single but may be multiple if the injury mechanism is repetitive in nature. For the same reason one or all nails may be involved. Aggressive removal of cuticle resulting in injuries to the proximal nail fold may result in the production of these lines. Repetitive minor shoe trauma to one or all toenails may produce this disorder (Figure 5-27).

White Spots. White spots in the nail plate are the result of minor localized injuries to the matrix bed. Some call this disorder "punctate leukonychia." They are seen more often in the fingernails than in toenails. Depending on the injury they vary from 1 to 3 mm in diameter. Some of the spots disappear before reaching the free edge of the nail. They cause no problems or symptoms.

Apparent Leukonychia. As touched on previously, apparent leukonychia is a condition of the underlying tissues. The nail plate is not white but only appears so. The most common cause of this in toenails is onycholysis of the nail plate from the nail bed. The light refracted through the plate when this disorder is present makes it appear white. Fungal infections of the nail bed and injury to the nail commonly produce this disorder (Figure 5-28).

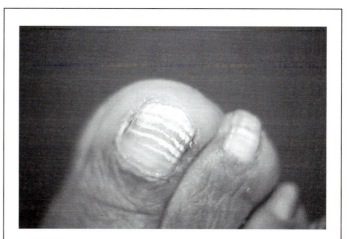

Figure 5-27 *Transverse leukonychia or leukonychia striata. This patient had this condition on both great toes and to a lesser extent on the second toes. It tends to have the shape of the proximal nail fold and the discoloration is in the plate. It may be caused from short shoes.*

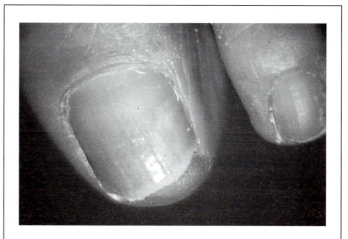

Figure 5-28 *The whitish area at the distal margin of this nail is caused by onycholysis of the plate from the underlying nail bed. This area refracts the light differently than the attached portions of the plate and makes the nail appear white. When the plate is compressed onto the nail bed the plate has a more normal appearance. In this case the condition is caused by a fungal infection of the nail bed.*

Melanonychia. This refers to black or brown discoloration in the nail. We have already discussed malignant melanoma, longitudinal melanonychia, splinter and subungual hemorrhage, and certain fungal infections as causes of this condition. Some nail enamels and hardeners may turn the surface of the nails a brownish or yellowish color. In toenails particularly, aging process and lack of proper care will turn the surface of the nail plate a brownish color. A *Proteus* bacterial infection, fairly common under toenails, will result in a gray to black discoloration in the infected area.

Yellow Discolorations. Yellow discolorations of the nail may occur as the result of the aging process. **Acquired Immunodeficiency Syndrome** (AIDS) may result in a yellowing of the nails. Some species of fungi turn the nail yellow in the affected areas. An infection under the plate resulting in the formation of a pus pocket will have a typical whitish-yellow appearance. The so-called yellow nail syndrome is characterized by a diffuse yellowish discoloration of all the nail plates that are also thickened and excessively curved from side to side. A slow growth of the nail plate, absence of the lunula and cuticle, swelling of the tissues around the nail, and in some cases variable degrees of onycholysis are also part of this syndrome. Various lung disorders such as emphysema, tuberculosis, asthma, and chronic bronchitis can cause this disorder. Other diseases also related to this syndrome include malignancies, rheumatoid arthritis, and thyroid disease.

Green Discolorations. These are usually the result of a disorder under the nail plate. *Pseudomonas* infections are probably the most common cause of this color change. *Aspergillus* species commonly found associated with fungal infections of the nail may appear as a green discoloration under the nail plate. A hematoma, if it has been present for some time under the nail, may take on a greenish-yellow color.

Red Discolorations. These also are usually the result of a soft tissue disorder under the nail plate. Subungual hematomas and splinter hemorrhages in their early formation stages will appear red in color. Congestive heart failure will cause the lunula to appear red. Rheumatoid arthritis when affecting the nail bed will cause it to appear red. The "oil drop" sign of the nail bed associated with psoriasis also appears as a reddish brown discoloration.

Bluish Discolorations. Blue discolorations of the nail results from subungual tissue disorders. Cyanosis or lack of oxygen in the blood is seen as a blue discoloration of the nail bed. This condition is often seen in individuals who have chronic obstructive lung disease. Early injuries to the nail such as those produced by improperly fit shoes are seen as a bluish discoloration of the nail bed.

Yellow nail syndrome is characterized by a diffuse yellowish discoloration of all the nail plates.

FOOT NOTES

This chapter has discussed the normal nail and disorders associated with the nail. The importance of understanding what makes up the normal components of the nail module cannot be overstressed. Without a full and complete understanding of how the normal nail plate is produced, it is impossible to understand or determine the causes of the various nail disorders. Too many times we look at the nail plate as an entity unto itself. We fail to recognize that the disorder or malformation we are observing is the result of a problem totally unrelated to what we are actually seeing. For these reasons the most important section of this chapter is "The Normal Nail!"

QUESTIONS

1. What are the six basic structures which compose the normal nail module?

2. Why is it important to understand how a normal nail is formed?

3. What does onychopathy mean?

4. What is the most common disorder of the toenails?

5. What are the most common nail plate deformities seen with an "ingrown nail?"

6. Should the nail professional trim back the edge of a plicatured deformity of the toenail?

7. What percent of the black population over the age of 50 have longitudinal melanonychia?

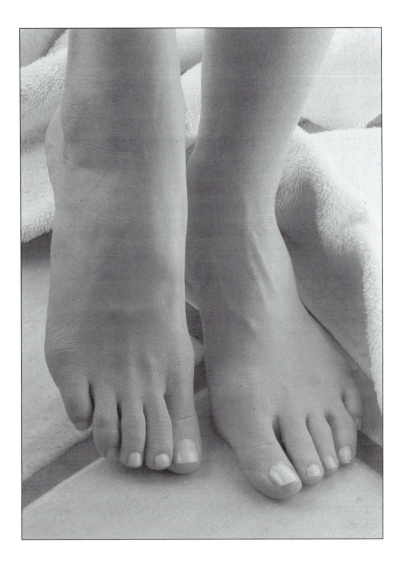

Foot Anomalies, Genetic and Medical | 6

LEARNING OBJECTIVES

After studying this chapter, the reader should be able to:

1. *Define anomaly and distinguish between a genetic and medical anomaly.*

2. *Briefly describe the types of syndactyly.*

3. *Define brachymetapody.*

4. *Define onychotillomania.*

An anomaly is a deviation from the average or norm. The dictionary defines the term as "anything that is structurally unusual or irregular or contrary to a general rule." An example of a **genetic** anomaly would be a congenital defect such as a cleft palate or in the foot, webbed toes. A medical anomaly may be many different things but in general is the result of a nongenetic medical condition such as the surgical loss of a toe. For purposes of this chapter the "structurally unusual or irregular" part of the definition applies.

— **L.O. 1**

HISTORY

In ancient times physical anomalies were thought to be a work of the devil or an omen sent from the gods. Physically deformed babies were often killed because of these beliefs. A physically deformed child in the house may cast an evil spell over the entire family. Societies eventually became more understanding and compassionate. However, individuals with physical deformities were still not truly accepted. Those who had them were shunned and kept out of view. Unscrupulous individuals, capitalizing on the morbid curiosity of society, opened "freak shows" charging the public to view the unusual human creations of nature.

It was not until the early 20th century that the science of genetics began evolving at a much faster pace. Serious scientific answers began to explain the causes of different inherited deformities and individual characteristics observed in the human population. Those with structurally unusual characteristics were no longer "freaks of nature." It was now understood that through no fault of their own they inherited these characteristics from their ancestors. This chapter discusses and shows a few of the genetic and medical anomalies that may on occasion be seen by those who work with the feet.

GENETIC ANOMALIES

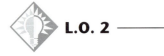

L.O. 2

Figure 6-1—This shows a partial **syndactyly** (webbing) (sin-dak'ti-le) of the second and third toes. This is the most common area of occurrence in the foot. The condition can usually be found in each generation of a family. This condition is usually not painful. Surgical reduction of syndactyly is usually performed for cosmetic reasons only.

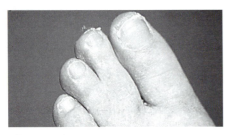

Figure 6-1

Figure 6-2—Double toenail. This is a fifth toe. Notice how wide the toe is compared to normal. There are two separate nail plates. This is the result of a full syndactyly of the fifth toe to an accessory sixth toe. The medical term for this condition is **synpolydactyly** (sin'pol-e-dak'ti-le). This condition does not bother the individual.

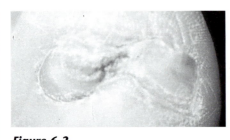

Figure 6-2

Figure 6-3—This shows a genetic condition in which the fifth toe overlaps the fourth toe. The medical name for this condition is "digiti quinti varus." The condition is usually not symptomatic. It can cause problems in wearing shoes and a surgical procedure can easily correct it.

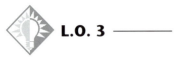

L.O. 3

Figure 6-4—This demonstrates a congenital shortening of the fourth ray (fourth metatarsal and phalanges). It is usually genetic in origin but can be caused from a childhood injury to the growth plate of the fourth metatarsal bone. It may occur in any of the metatarsals but the fourth is the most common. The medical term for this condition is **brachymetapody** (brak'e-me-tap'o-de).

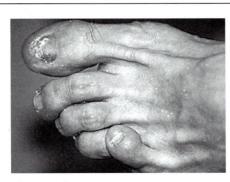

Figure 6-3

Figure 6-5—This is an x-ray of the foot seen in the Figure 6-4. Notice the extremely short fourth metatarsal although the toe is normally formed. This condition generally

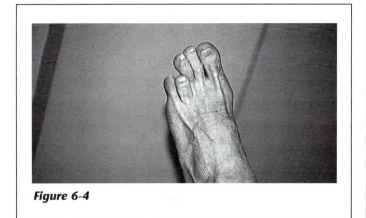

Figure 6-4

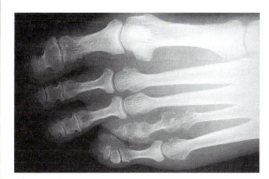

Figure 6-5

does not cause symptoms. Younger individuals may want it corrected for cosmetic reasons. This can be accomplished; however, the procedure is expensive and complicated. It is difficult to lengthen the small blood vessels to the toe. The stretching of the vessels may cause a blockage, which leads to gangrene, and a resultant loss of the toe may be a complication of the procedure.

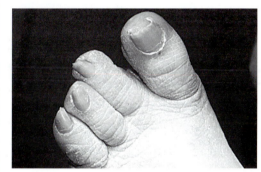

Figure 6-6

Figure 6-6—This photograph shows the congenital absence of the entire fifth ray (fifth metatarsal and phalanges). The foot looks absolutely normal with the exception of there being no fifth toe. This lady was born with this condition on only one foot. To make her feet appear normal her parents had the fifth ray of the other foot amputated when she was 12 years old. Both feet now look identical and one has to look twice to see that there is an anomaly present. In this case, therefore, one foot is a genetic and the other is a medical anomaly.

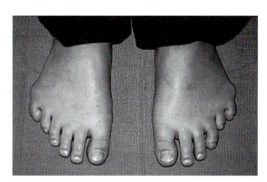

Figure 6-7

Figure 6-7—This condition is the opposite of that in Figure 6-6. In this case the individual was born with six toes on both feet. The medical term for this condition is **polydactyly** (pol-e-dak'ti-le). Previous generations of the family also had this condition. The patient sought removal of the accessory digits because her shoes were painful as a result of the very prominent metatarsal heads.

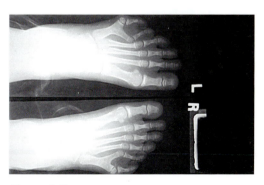

Figure 6-8

Figure 6-8—This is an x-ray of the feet showing the Y-shaped fifth metatarsal and extra toe.

L.O. 4 — **Figure 6-9**—This elderly lady was referred because of a complaint of fungus in her nails. On examination all of her toenails were picked down to the nail beds. Most of the nail plates were totally gone with a raw nail bed being visible. Some of them even had fresh dried blood around and over the nail beds! This lady had the pathologic habit of picking her nails and used her impression of a fungus to excuse this habit. The medical name for this condition is **onychotillomania** (on,i-kot'i-lo-ma'ne-a), defined as a tendency to pick at the nails.

Figure 6-10 —This is a view of the left thumb of the lady with onychotillomania. All of the nails on her left hand looked this severe if not worse. The nails on her right hand were absolutely normal! This lady only picked at her nails, she was not a nail biter. The nails on her left hand were so short she could not use them to pick at the nails on her right hand!

Figure 6-11—This lady was seen for a problem other than the large black area of skin on her heel. On first look this area had the appearance of a large melanoma. On closer examination the edges appeared to be scarred. It seems she had a previous injury to her heel, which resulted in a full thickness loss of skin at that site. This required skin grafting to repair the defect. Because she was black and the graft came from her thigh, which was much darker than her heel, the dark area surrounded by a lighter colored skin was the result.

Figure 6-12—This patient came in for routine maintenance of her nails. She has always had this large, toe-like, mass between her first and second toes. It is about half the size of her great toe! It does not hurt and she says she has had it since she was a young girl. It is firm and

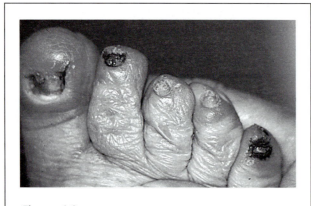

Figure 6-9

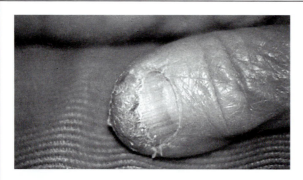

Figure 6-10

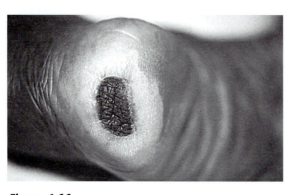

Figure 6-11

appears to have many large and small blood vessels within it. For this reason it is called a **telangiectatic** fibroma (tel-an'je-ek-tat'ik, fi-bro'ma) or a fibrous tumor filled with blood vessels. It may be related to a type of a birthmark.

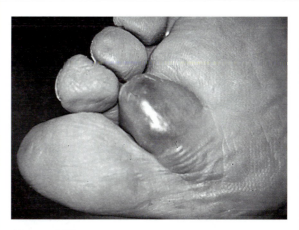

Figure 6-12

FOOT NOTES

Nature works in mysterious ways. From Chapter 1 we have seen how the human foot evolved to what we now know. Who is to say that at one time our foot was not an anomaly when it first began to evolve? We now look on the "flat foot" as an anomaly but 1.75 million years ago it was the norm. Who are we five-toed individuals to say that six or four toes are an anomaly? Maybe 1.75 million years from now four-toed, or will it be six-toed, *Homo sapiens* will be the norm. Contemplate this when you see someone who, at least at this period of evolution, deviates from the average or norm as you compare their physical form to your own!

QUESTIONS

1. What is an anomaly?

2. What is onychotillomania?

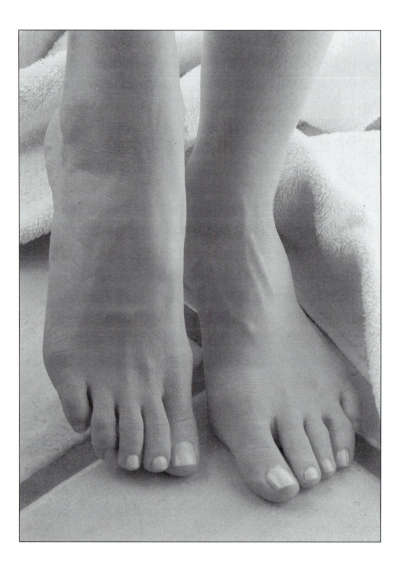

Client
History 7

LEARNING OBJECTIVES

After studying this chapter, the reader should be able to:

1. *Discuss the importance of the first contact with a new client.*

2. *Describe the setting for an effective client interview.*

3. *List the information obtained by using the new client encounter form.*

4. *Explain the difference between a client's chronologic and physiologic age.*

5. *List the information obtained by using the medical history form.*

6. *Discuss what is involved in the personal evaluation of a new client.*

GENERAL OVERVIEW

Although this book is about the foot and its care, this chapter should be the foundation for evaluating any new client for services within the beauty industry. In the litigious society in which we live, the importance of keeping proper client records cannot be overstressed. By learning the principles of history taking you will be able to serve your clients' needs in an enhanced professional manner. Through a series of questions you will be able to determine allergies, illnesses, medications, needs, and likes and dislikes of your new client. This should not be a long, involved process. You need to practice and modify your technique to enable you to ask questions and elicit information in an orderly and timely manner. If done properly these questions will not make clients feel you are prying into their business or personal affairs. You will find that as you become more proficient in this process a few well thought out questions will elicit most of the necessary information you need. If people are relaxed and at ease in their surroundings they like nothing better than to talk about them-

The importance of keeping proper client records cannot be overstressed.

selves. You will find that once the proper question is asked all you will need to do is sit back and become a good listener. The art of the process comes in being able to direct the discussion to where you want it to go.

L.O. 1

Your initial contact with new clients, as well as theirs with you, will be the basis for all future interactions between you. This is the time when mutual respect is developed. Clients are determining whether they will be satisfied with your services. You are determining whether you will be able to satisfy their needs as they perceive them. You both are determining whether this will be a good or bad relationship, all based on first impressions. It is important for you as a business professional, rendering personal services, to learn all you can about new clients and not let your individual perceptions cloud your judgments.

The new client has already made a decision to seek your services based on a number of factors. A satisfied client referral, location, availability, work hours, and reputation are some of the factors that have helped the person choose you. It is now up to you to show that she has made the right choice. Sitting down with her in a personal friendly manner and discussing her wants, needs, and expectations will start this process. Be yourself! If you are too formal and businesslike you may inhibit the ability to communicate. On the other hand, a casual attitude will fail to instill confidence. Avoid extremes in your reactions to answers elicited by your questions. Overreaction to a question may be interpreted by the client as lack of understanding or caring on your part. Be a good listener as well as a good **facilitator** and **communicator** and you will maintain a satisfying long-lasting professional relationship.

Being a good facilitator and communicator will enhance your relationships with clients.

Your primary objective during this initial consultation is to find out what services the client desires from you and to do something about it. You need to identify the client's underlying worries, believe them no matter how trivial, and suggest services that will work within their setting. Secondarily, a general understanding of the client's medical history will enhance your ability to recommend safe products and services. You need to specifically understand what that client expects from you. If expectations are too high or beyond your capabilities discuss this in detail so there is an understanding about what you can deliver. If you know that the client's expectations are unobtainable be frank and try to assist her in lowering these expectations to more reasonable levels. If this then is still not satisfactory assist the client in trying to obtain the desired services from someone else. You may be pleasantly surprised when that client returns for the service you recommended in the first place.

Remember, first impressions usually will govern all future interactions in any relationship whether it be professional or personal. Each time you walk into your salon enter it as if you were entering it for the first time. Look around and see it as if you were looking through the eyes of a new client. Is it clean, neat, and a place where you would like to have personal services rendered to you? If not, change it! Otherwise when you later are developing a relationship with your new client, her mind will still be out in the reception area thinking about the dirty rug or cracked mirror that made her wonder if she had made the right choice in seeking out your services. It is imperative that you have her undivided attention at this critical point in developing your future professional relationship with her.

Take client histories somewhere other than at your work table. The ideal would be in a place where your products are displayed so that you may discuss the individual products that you will recommend for care. This area should be well-lighted, furnished with comfortable chairs, a small uncluttered work table or desk as well as a stool the client can put her foot on if she is there for a pedicure. This surrounding should make the client feel relaxed and it will allow her to open up to you regarding her needs and expectations for the services desired. In this surrounding you will be able to ask questions and get answers more easily than in an open public area.

——— **L.O. 2**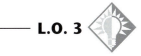

INITIAL ENCOUNTER FORM

This is the form the client should fill out when being seen for their first appointment. It will give you basic information that will allow you to set up your record file and it also helps you begin the history-taking process. If the proper data are on this form, the information will help you formulate questions to ask during the history portion of this visit (Figure 7-1).

This form will be slightly different for each individual salon. Start with a basic format and modify it for your individual needs. If you find part of it does not work for you, change it! Make it work for you as well as the client.

This form should elicit the following information:

Accurate information on your clients is invaluable and will not require much time to obtain.

1. *Name and address (home and work).* This is a basic. From the addresses you will be able to determine demographics of your clients. This will assist in advertising or promoting services. If you find your clients are coming from one particular area you may advertise more heavily in those areas than others. Or vice versa. It can also tell you a little about the financial background of the client.

——— **L.O. 3**

2. *Telephone numbers (home, work, pager, etc.).* Also another basic. This allows you to communicate with your clients. You can confirm appointments or if you need to reschedule them because you are ill or running behind they may be easily reached. As you are well

New Client Encounter Form

Name: _____   Birth Date: ___ / ___ / ___

Address: _____   Phone (daytime) _____

City _____ State _____ Zip _____   Phone (evening) _____

Occupation _____   Pager/FAX _____

Previous Services: Pedicures ☐   Manicures ☐   Hot paraffin wax
                         Reflexology ☐   Other ☐   (feet/hands) ☐

Artificial Nails: Acrylic ☐   Fiberglass/Silk ☐   Other ☐

Any allergic reactions to beauty products?   Yes ☐   No ☐

If yes, please explain: _____

_____

Any special skin or nail problems? _____

_____

Who referred you to our salon?

Phone book ☐   Location ☐   Friend ☐   Self ☐   Other ☐

☐ One of our clients (name) _____

Signature _____

Date: ____ / ____ / ____

Figure 7-1 *This is the suggested format for a client initial encounter form. It may need to be modified for your use. The client should fill out this form and sign it.*

aware there are many different reasons why you may need to contact them!

3. *Birthday.* This gives the age of the client. More than that you should use it to determine **chronologic** versus **physiologic** age of the client. You have seen people who "do not look their age," meaning they either look older or younger than they actually are. If a person is 50 years old but looks 65 or 70 years old then her chronologic age is younger than the physiologic age. With this type of client you will have to be much more careful than someone who is 70 but appears to be 55 or 60. A person who is aging faster than the actual, or chronologic age, may be one who is more prone to medical problems, circulatory disorders, or infections. Learn to recognize these clients and recommend services that will fit their individual needs.

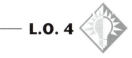
—— **L.O. 4**

4. *Occupation.* This will tell you a lot about your clients. Their work is really a mirror on their life. Does their job require them to be on their feet for long hours? What type of footgear do they wear— rubber boots, pumps, flats, athletic style shoes? Each of these can cause different problems. Are their hands or feet constantly exposed to harsh materials or moisture? Different products will work better for these individuals than if they were typists or accountants. Learn to fit the service to the demands of the client's occupation.

Learn to fit the service to the demands of the client's occupation.

5. *What previous professional nail services have you had?* Here you may want to list the various services most commonly provided. Manicures, pedicures, overlays, wraps, reflexology, and so on. What you are trying to determine is what they are familiar with, whether they were happy with those services, and if not why not? This question opens the door for other discussions about previous experiences, bad or good, with professional nail services and personnel. It will keep you from repeating past bad experiences this client may have been exposed to in another setting.

6. *Have you ever had, or thought you have had, a reaction to a beauty product?* You may wish to list things such as acetone, polish removers, acrylic compounds, fiberglass, and so forth. This question will save headaches in your future care of this client. Again you do not want to create a bad situation that would be a repeat of the client's past. In general, each subsequent reaction to an irritant is worse than the previous one. A patient who was allergic to adhesive tape was seen after his first reaction and advised not to allow anyone to put adhesive tape on him again. The next week he was seen again, only this time he was in the hospital with his foot swollen, red, and weeping fluid from blisters where he had allowed another doctor to reapply adhesive tape to his foot. He had forgotten to tell the doctor about his tape allergy! This is extreme but as you see it can happen. By getting the client to answer this question in writing you are also helping to relieve yourself from liability if your client reacts to something he did not tell you about.

7. *Who referred you for my services?* You may wish to make this a checklist: friend, another client, telephone book, location, other. If it was another client you should find out the name so you can thank that client, but more importantly it also gives hints as to what this client wants. Generally friends refer friends for similar services. This also helps you find out if your ads in the telephone book or other promotions you may be doing are working. If no one is coming because of your ad in the telephone book you may want to redo it in a different style next year.

Be sure to thank those who have referred new clients to you.

CLIENT MEDICAL HISTORY

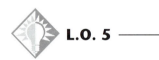

L.O. 5 ——— This form (Figure 7-2) can be used when you start talking with the client about medical history. It is a cursory history that will allow you to get to know your client's general medical background and to recommend appropriate services.

1. *What is the name of your primary care doctor? Do you see a podiatrist or dermatologist? What are their names?* It is important to know what doctors your client sees. It gives you another insight on this client. More importantly if this client should ever develop a medical problem that may be related to your services you can communicate with the doctor and discuss it. It makes it easier to refer the client to the doctor if the need arises. If there is ever a question as to whether your service is causing a medical problem for the client, it is much better for you to voice your professional concern to the doctor and client than to have the client go to the doctor on her own. The client will appreciate your professional concern and recognition of the condition. The doctor will appreciate the fact that you are a knowledgeable professional in your field who is concerned about your client's well-being. You may have to explain to clients why you need to know the names of their doctors. Approach this directly and tell them you are concerned with their

Client Medical History

Birth Date: ___ / ___ / ___

Name of your primary care physician _____

Name of your podiatrist _____

Name of your dermatologist _____

List any medications you are currently taking: _____

_____

List any medical problems: _____

_____

List any food or drug allergies: _____

_____

Figure 7-2 *This is a suggested client medical history and personal evaluation form to be filled out by the nail professional during the client's initial appointment.*

health as it relates to your services. Advise them that under no circumstances would you contact the doctor without first discussing it with them and obtaining their permission. You need to do this so clients do not feel that you may go behind their back and discuss their private matters with someone.

2. *Do you take any medications?* Here again you will want to make a list of some medications that are known to cause disorders of the nails or skin. What medications an individual takes will tell you a lot about that person's health. If the client takes insulin or an oral medication such as DiaBeta you will know immediately this individual is a diabetic. A good reference book for the salon is "PDR, Physicians Desk Reference,"published by Medical Economics Company. This book lists all the prescription medications on the market. Indications (what the medication is used for), side effects, contraindications, and a vast amount of other information are listed for each medication. At first the amount of information may

seem overwhelming but you will find that a few medications are commonly used and you will become easily acquatinted with their names.

Medical conditions in your clients can affect your services.

3. *Are you being treated for any medical problems?* The main problems you will be interested in, particularly when it comes to the foot, are those relating to the circulatory system, diabetes, and skin conditions. A checklist of the medical problems that will most affect your services is an easy quick method of obtaining a response to this question. Certain medical conditions can be directly related to your care. You will need to be much more conservative and gentle in giving a pedicure service to someone with psoriasis, diabetes, or poor circulation. Clients with skin problems will need special attention when you recommend different skin care products. Clients with other conditions such as rheumatoid arthritis will require special services to make them as comfortable as possible in the salon setting.

4. *Do you have any allergies to foods or drugs?* Here you are looking for general information on this subject. Certain beauty products on the market may have egg or vegetable bases in them. It is nice to know if the client is allergic to things such as this. It will help you make product recommendations for their future care. Some individuals seem to be allergic to everything. These clients require conservative care. Try different products one at a time to see if the client has any adverse reactions to them. The knowledge of any allergies the client may have can greatly enhance your ability to render professional services.

This gives a general outline for a basic initial encounter form. Once the client has filled it out you need to sit down and discuss it with her in the surroundings previously discussed. Verify information and obtain more in-depth information in those areas that might affect the particular services you will recommend for the client. This will be particularly important in clients who have diabetes, skin conditions, or circulatory problems. Medical conditions in your clients can affect your services and whether you should provide services for them at all.

PERSONAL EVALUATION

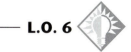 L.O. 6

After completing the history portion of the initial visit it is then time to do a personal evaluation of the client (Figure 7-3). This is where you will actually examine the client both visually and by touch. How in-depth this evaluation will be depends on what you have discovered in the history and what services the client desires. This evaluation should be done by any beauty professional before giving hair, skin, or nail services. You should keep a written record of your findings for future reference. It will allow you to determine if the conditions you observe are new or were present previously. For the purpose of this book we will discuss the evaluation of the foot and lower extremity. A similar evaluation can be done for beauty services given in areas other than the foot.

During your previous discussion with the client you should have already determined whether she appears older, younger, or about the stated age. From this you will already have some insight about the physical status of the client. Have the client remove her shoes and hosiery. First look at the foot and leg as one. Are there any deformities—webbed toes, missing toes, one leg shorter than the other? Is any swelling present in the foot, around the ankles, or in the legs? If so is it in both legs or feet, in one more than the other, or only on one side?

Check the circulation by feeling the pulses in the foot. To render a safe pedicure service one should at least be able to feel (palpate) these pulses. They are located on the top of the foot and behind and under the medial malleolus (see Chapter 2). Also check the capillary filling time in the toes. This is done by pressing on the skin over the distal end of the toe and then releasing the pressure. The area of tissue that was under pressure will be white or blanched out because the blood was squeezed out of the capillaries. The time it takes for the blood to return to the area, which is indicated by the tissues becoming pink again, is called the **capillary filling time**. For the purpose of this book this time should be less than 30 seconds.

The skin should be evaluated next. Is it normal texture and temperature or dry and scaly, shiny and tight? Is there normal hair growth or no hair growth at all? Are there any corns or calluses or other skin lesions such as apparent infections, nevi (moles), ulcers, or bruises? Are there any fungal infections (athlete's foot) between the toes or on other areas of the foot or leg? What do the nails look like? Are they normal thickness and color? Are they incurvated or ingrown? Do any of the nails have an apparent fungal infection? Do they cause pain or discomfort; if so, what type of pain or discomfort? Is the pain, sharp, dull, or throbbing? When does the pain occur? At night, when walking, or when wearing shoes?

Your evaluation of a client should be kept in a written record so you have it for future reference.

Personal Evaluation

Birth Date: ___ / ___ / ___

Hands/Fingernails

Condition of fingernails, cuticles, and skin: _____

_____

Legs/Feet/Toenails

Deformities: _____

Swelling: _____

Circulation/Pulses: DP ☐   PT ☐ Capillary filling time: _____

Condition of skin:

Thin ☐   Dry ☐   Shiny ☐   Scaly ☐ Cracked ☐ Normal ☐

☐ Other_____

Skin lesions (corns/calluses/nevi/ulcers/etc.): _____

_____

_____

Infections (fungal/other): _____

_____

_____

Description of nails (color, shape, ingrown, thickness, infections, etc.): _____

_____

_____

Figure 7-3 *Personal evaluation form*

Now let us discuss what we are learning from the above evaluation. By first looking at the general appearance of the foot and leg you are again determining physiologic versus chronologic age. It can give you an idea as to whether the client is taking care of the lower extremities. If not why not? Can she not see or reach her feet? Is she merely neglecting them? It is important to know the difference! If clients are neglecting them for no reason, you may find they will not follow the instructions you give them for the use of products you may recommend.

General physical deformities may be a determining factor in the services and products you recommend. Swelling (edema) is an important finding. Pitting edema is a condition that when pressure is applied to the swollen part there will be left a persistent depression or "pit" in the affected tissues after the pressure is released. The depth of the depression is a measurement of the severity of the swelling and is recorded in the records as 1+, 2+, 3+, and 4+ pitting edema. 1+ is a very superficial depression, and 4+ is a much deeper depression and indicates much more swelling. Heart, kidney, and vascular problems at times manifest first in the feet or lower extremity. Lower extremity surgeries, infections, injuries and poor **lymphatic** drainage can also cause swelling in the feet and legs. In a few instances hereditary factors can cause lower extremity edema.

General physical deformities may be a determining factor in the services and products you recommend.

As a general rule if the swelling is not present in the morning when the client arises from bed it is nothing to worry about. In these cases it may be termed dependent edema or swelling caused only because of the pooling of fluid in the lowest part of the body. If the swelling is present in the morning the same as it was the night before it is generally caused by a disease process. You should question the client about how long the swelling has been present. Swelling that has been present for a long while is usually being looked after by the physician or may be a normal condition for that particular individual. Swelling that has not been present for any length of time may indicate the onset of a more severe problem. Also ask whether the client has been short of breath during normal walking or when climbing stairs. A yes answer may indicate a heart condition and you should suggest an early visit to the doctor for a physical examination. Your suggestion may well save the client from more severe problems in the future. Swelling in only one leg (unilateral) may be caused from a blockage in the lymphatics or venous blood system on that side. Long-standing edematous conditions cause the lymphatic vessels and tissue spaces to be stretched to the point where they will never return to their normal size. The resultant condition is called chronic edema. In this condition one may see changes in the skin, one of which can be a roughened "orange peel" texture. The massage and skin services of the pedicure should be very gentle so as not to cause injury to the already stretched and irritated skin.

While checking the circulation you can begin checking the condition of the skin. Dry scaly skin along with the absence of hair growth in the lower extremity usually can be associated with poor circulation. Shiny tight skin can also be associated with a poor circulatory status. Dependent rubor or cyanosis (conditions in which the lower leg and foot exhibit red or blue color changes if the foot is on the floor) indicates fairly advanced vascular disease. You will need to correlate these skin findings with your evaluation of the pulses and capillary filling time to help confirm if a poor circulatory status exists.

Infections or open sores will indicate that a pedicure service should not be performed until they are resolved or healed. A referral to the podiatrist or dermatologist for treatment is indicated here. Fungal infections (athlete's foot), if not open and bleeding, do not necessarily rule out a pedicure service. For this personal evaluation part of the service it is necessary to determine the presence of the fungus, its severity, and its location. If it is severe with blisters, moist areas, or large areas of red irritated skin, a medical referral before performing a pedicure service is indicated. Clients with minor long-standing fungal infections can safely receive a pedicure service if standard disinfectant precautions are followed before and after the service is performed.

Infections or open sores will indicate that a pedicure service should not be performed until they are resolved or healed.

The location and size of nevi should be recorded. By keeping a record, any change in size or color will be easier to recognize during future pedicure services. Any nevus that does not look right to you should be referred for a medical checkup. It is better to have 10 normal checkups than to miss one melanoma!

The nails, which will be your primary concern, should be evaluated closely. A statement about the general appearance of the nails in most cases will be adequate: "Normal incurvation, thickness, and color with no abnormal growth patterns noted." If any abnormal conditions are seen such as thickening, ingrowing, discolorations, or fungus, the condition should be noted and which nails are involved. It is helpful to record how long the condition has been present. This can give an insight as to the possible cause. The client should be asked whether the condition is uncomfortable or not. If the answer is yes the next thing to learn is what type of discomfort the client is feeling. Different types of pain—sharp, stabbing, aching, burning, throbbing—are generally associated with different conditions. Throbbing pain is generally associated with an infection; an aching pain is generally caused by pressure. What causes the pain to start also gives an idea as to what abnormal condition is the cause. If it only hurts in shoes in all probability the shoe is the causative factor. If there is discomfort walking as well as resting, or wearing shoes or not wearing shoes, an acute condition such as an infection should be suspected.

At first you may ask why you need to know the information that has been discussed. The answer is whatever you do to the client will affect the entire individual. All of these questions will give you an important insight into your new client's general foot health and over all well-being. The more you know about the client will allow you to provide professional quality services. You will be able to tailor your services for that individual so they will be beneficial and not cause harm.

This procedure will in most instances be short and not involved. A young healthy individual does not require the time it will take for someone who has more complicated physical problems. It is important for you to recognize the difference and tailor the depth of personal evaluation for the individual client. This does not mean that the process of the evaluation should be skipped. The actual steps performed will be the same for everyone.

Whatever you do to your client will affect the entire person.

FOOT NOTES

The initial client visit sets the stage for all future professional relationships that you will have with a client. It is the one and only time you will have to make a first impression on that client. Make the most of it! Develop an expertise in the manner in which you ask questions and direct a conversation. Lead your client into the conversation you desire. Avoid overreacting to a client's answers. Remember you are the professional and a caring non-judgmental demeanor will impart this to the client. Your time is valuable—you do not want to waste it on small talk, particularly at this time. Educate your clients on the reasons why you are asking about their medical history. Become a good listener!

QUESTIONS

1. Why is the initial encounter form important?

2. Why is it important for you to know about any previous allergies the client may have had?

3. Why is it important for you to know about the client's medical history?

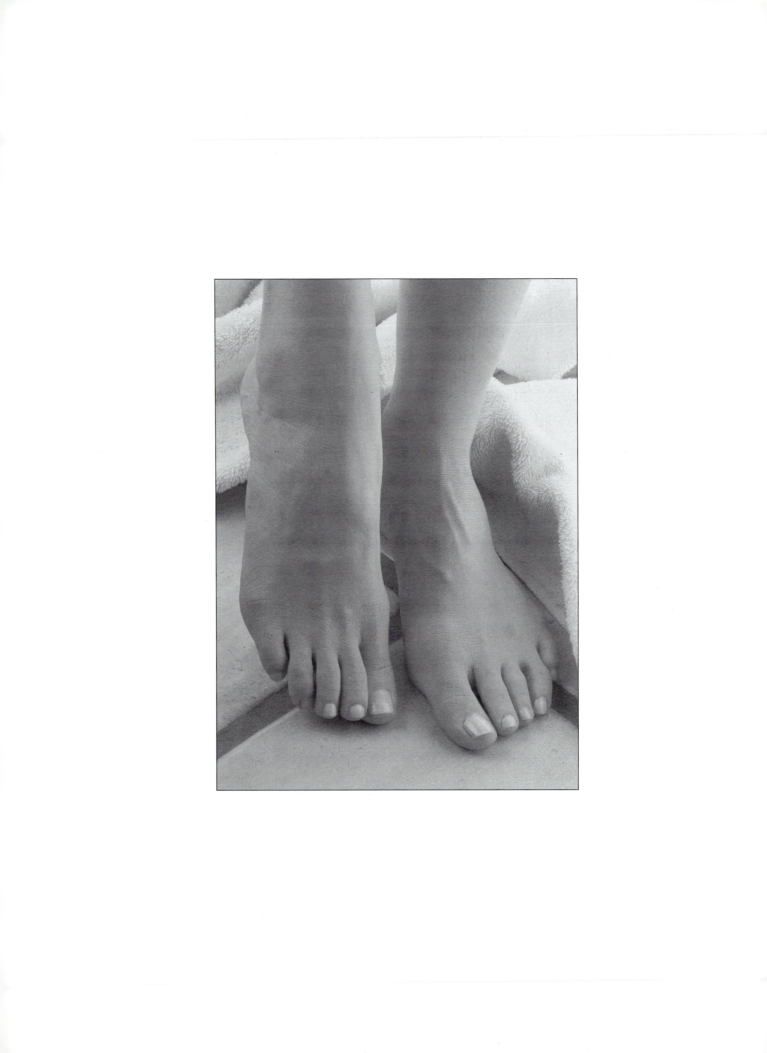

Instruments and Equipment | 8

LEARNING OBJECTIVES

After studying this chapter, the reader should be able to:

1. *Discuss the reasons for purchasing quality instruments.*

2. *Describe the five basic instruments for providing foot services, including their specific uses.*

3. *Describe an ingrown nail shaver and a cuticle nipper and their use.*

4. *Describe the four types of drills used in providing foot services.*

5. *Discuss the different types of drill bits and their uses.*

6. *Describe, compare, and contrast the various types of salon equipment— carts, water baths, and spas.*

GENERAL DISCUSSION

It cannot be stressed enough that the nail professional must use quality professional instruments and equipment in the performance of client services. The word professional is defined as "having or showing great skill; or an expert." Each profession has tools or equipment specific to that particular profession. These tools allow professionals to perform their skills in a skilled manner. How many times have you heard, "The right tools make the job easy." This is particularly true when it comes to working on the foot. I was a new member on a hospital staff and was doing one of my first foot surgeries in the operating room of that hospital. I had practiced at other hospitals that had the proper instruments and assumed that this hospital would have similar or like equipment for me to use. How wrong I was! They had previously done little foot surgery in this hospital. When I asked for a **pneumatic** bone saw I was given a very large pneumatic saw, over a foot long, which was used for cutting much larger bone. In trying to make it work on the foot I **contaminated** the end of it when it touched my chin while I was sawing. The surgery had to be stopped while the saw was resterilized. This added an extra 15 minutes to the surgery time and, needless to say, the great embarrassment I experienced while waiting. The surgery turned out well but next time I did surgery at that hospital I made sure the **micro** saw, which is about 6 inches in length and half the diameter of the other saw, was available for my use.

Improper instruments used in the performance of foot services by the nail professional can easily cause injury to toenails and the soft tissues of the foot. The use of proper instruments and equipment is therefore a major requirement in providing quality professional foot services to your clients. Instruments and equipment made for the express purpose of working on the feet will allow the nail professional to provide a safer service to clients. Proper instruments and equipment will make the provision of foot services easier and quicker. Thus, providing foot services becomes a much more pleasant experience for the nail professional as well as for the client. This chapter will assist you in selecting the proper instruments and equipment to provide these services.

Improper instruments can easily cause injury to toenails and the soft tissues of the foot.

There are very few quality instruments for foot care being sold to the nail professional. What are being provided are totally inadequate, unsafe, or cheap imitations of the types of instruments that should be used for foot care. Distributors do not really know how the instrument should be used on the foot so they cannot demonstrate its use properly. In their defense they should not have to do this. The schools should be doing this but in most instances they are not. As usual, the foot seems to be the last thing on the list to be discussed during the educational process. This is not unusual. It happens even in medical schools!

Most distributors say that the nail professional will not pay the price for a quality professional instrument. If this is true it is because no one has ever taken the time to explain to the nail professional what or why particular instruments should be used to provide foot services. Nor does the nail professional understand the cost effectiveness of quality instruments. Because of this, nail professionals remain ignorant, through no fault of their own, about what to purchase. A quality instrument will last the user many years and therefore becomes more cost effective than purchasing cheap instruments that will have to be replaced at regular intervals.

Nail professionals all wish to provide quality pedicure services but they have not been instructed how to use the proper instruments required for provision of these services. They have been trying to modify the use of the same instruments that they were taught to use on the hands. This is unsatisfactory and because of this they lose interest in providing pedicure services. They fail to promote these services as they should and thus a large part of their potential income is lost.

The hands and feet are different! Toenails are shaped differently than fingernails. Toenails have more side-to-side curve and are thicker than finger-nails. Therefore, modified fingernail clippers are totally inadequate for trimming toenails. The so-called podiatry toenail cutters or pedicure nail nipper seen on the market, and at the shows, have the same jaw shape as the large toenail clippers and are not best suited for trimming toenails. The same nail files used for fingernails are being used for toenails. Toenails have more fungal infections than fingernails. Because of their construction, these files cannot be properly disinfected. In reality they should only be used on a one-time basis. This is not cost effective. Instead you are being told to sanitize the file and put it in a plastic bag or box with the client's name on it. You are then told to use the file on that same client at the next appointment. Think about this— the enclosed bag or box is a perfect environment for promoting fungal and bacterial growth! What would you think of your doctor getting out a baggy with your name on it and using the same tongue depressor he had used on you at your last visit? This is absurd but is basically the same scenario as saving an individual client's instruments in a baggy or box. There is a better file and we will talk about it in this chapter.

Equipment for treating fingernails does not necessarily work for treating toenails.

Let's talk about the Credo® Blade. In California if a state inspector finds one in the salon it can be grounds for license suspension. Despite this, they are being sold at all of the trade shows. Remember, just because they are being sold does not make their use legal. More importantly their promotion as a callus cutter does not make them an instrument to be used on the foot. They appear to be a modified potato peeler! The Credo® Blade may be dangerous to the foot health of your clients and therefore should not be used on the foot. You will not see a podiatrist using this instrument. They all use a surgical blade made for the purpose of removing callus tissue. You may say "but my clients demand that I remove their calluses." If a client has enough callus to be removed with a sharp instrument then you need to educate her about seeing a podiatrist for such removal. The various callus files and abrasive creams used for pedicures will adequately smooth any callus that requires care by the nail professional.

It is not recommended to use a pumice or other abrasive stones that are promoted for removing callus tissue from the foot. They are impossible to properly clean and disinfect. The porous nature of the stone combined with the many holes and cracks fill up with callus debris. This debris cannot be properly removed from the stone, so it becomes a perfect medium for the growth of bacteria and fungi. Having a pumice stone for resale to individual clients for home use is acceptable. The client will be using the product only on herself, which eliminates the problem of the transmission of organisms to others. Be sure to advise clients not to remove too much of their callus when they use the stone. The formation of callus is for protection and if too much is removed the area will become more painful and sore than it was before the removal.

INSTRUMENTS

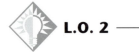

L.O. 2

Most of the instruments recommended in this section, or adaptations of them, are available from industry instrument suppliers (see Appendix for sources). Five basic instruments are recommended for providing foot services. These are the toenail nippers, a curette, a small nail rasp (file), a regular nail file, and a foot file or paddle. There is also a small ingrown nail shaver made for cutting the nail margins of the big toenails that on occasion is a useful and time-saving instrument. You should already have cuticle nippers for the fingers and the same ones can be used, if necessary, on the feet. All of these instruments except some of the foot paddles can be kept in a disinfecting solution 24 hours a day as long as there is an antirust inhibitor incorporated with the disinfectant. An electric drill is a time saver when it comes to thick toenails and you may also want to have this in your foot service area.

Quality instruments not only work better but will last longer and thus are quite cost effective. Remember this as you make your purchases and look for instruments that match or are as close to those pictured as possible. Now let us discuss the individual instruments and how to use them.

Know how to trim the toenail—one clip is not correct!

Toenail Nippers

Remember these are not the modified fingernail clippers! These are a professional instrument made for cutting bone or nails (Figure 8-1). They come with either curved or straight jaws. The long, slender, pointed jaws are the important thing to look for. The jaws of the nipper should come to a fairly fine point. Some come with a blunt point, which makes it very hard to trim out the small corners of a plicatured nail. Yes, in certain circumstances a small corner of the nail should be trimmed out! If done properly, trimming the corner of a toenail, which this nipper allows you to do, does not cause an ingrown toenail.

This instrument should be used like a pair of scissors. One should make a number of small cuts when cutting off the free edge of toenail. Toenails normally have more of a side-to-side curve than do fingernails. Do not try to clip the nail all the way across with one clip, which would flatten out the nail. This is painful or at the least uncomfortable for the client. More importantly, attempting to cut the free edge of the nail in one cut increases the probability of injuring the hyponychium or breaking its seal onto the nail plate. This makes a portal of entry for bacterial or fungal infections to occur under the nail. After trimming the nail for length, the fine point on the nipper can be used to trim out the small sharp point of nails that curve deeply into the nail margin (see Chapter 10).

The Curette

A **curette** is a small spoon-shaped instrument that allows for the removal of debris from the nail margins (Figures 8-2 and 8-3). Most curettes are quite sharp on their edges although others are dull. One recommendation may be a double-ended curette that has a 1.5-mm diameter curette on one end and a 2.5-mm diameter curette on the other. The curette should be small and not sharp. Some are made with a small hole in the curette and others do not have the hole. Some people find the ones with a hole easier to clean after they have been used. The curette for the purpose of nail care should not be used to cut out any tissue or debris along the nail margin. The nail professional must, for safety purposes, use a dull-edged curette.

To use this instrument place the rounded side of the spoon toward the living skin. This allows the edge of the instrument to fall against the side or edge of the nail. A scooping motion is then used along the nail plate to drag any loose debris or callus out of the nail groove. A gentle pressure against the nail plate and along the free edge of the nail margin is all that is necessary to accomplish the removal of the built up debris. The pressure of this debris is uncomfortable if left in place. You may need to repeat this scooping motion a number of times to adequately remove enough of the loose debris. WARNING: Do not use this instrument to dig into the soft tissues along the nail fold. These tissues are thin and may be easily injured. Any callus or other debris attached to the soft tissues that is not easily removed in the manner described should be removed by a podiatrist.

As you become proficient in the safe use of the curette you will find that it becomes

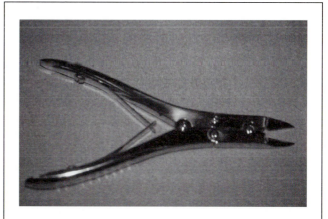

Figure 8-1 These are toenail nippers. These have a double action hinge and are easier to use than those with a single hinge. The slender pointed jaws are the key to allow proper trimming of toenails.

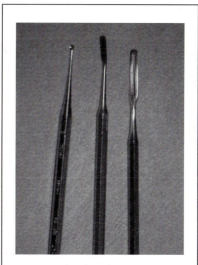

Figure 8-2 From left to right, curette, nail rasp, and ingrown nail shaver.

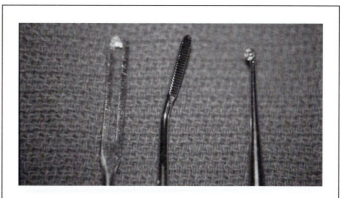

Figure 8-3 From left to right, a close up of the curette, nail rasp, and ingrown nail shaver.

an extension of the fingers in feeling for any rough edges or "hooks" that may have been left after the trimming process. Properly used the curette is the ideal instrument for cleaning the debris from and feeling along the nail margins. In most clients you will only have to use it along the margins of the great toenails. Only once in a while is it necessary to clean along the lesser toenail margins. These nails do not usually curve into the margin as much as the great toenail does and thus less debris builds up.

Nail Rasp or Small Nail File

This metal file, or rasp as it is called in the medical field, is constructed so that it only cuts or files in one direction (see Figures 8-2 and 8-3). The cutting part of the instrument is about one-eighth of an inch wide and about three-fourths of an inch long. It is attached to a metal handle in a straight or angled manner. The angled file can be easier to use along the nail groove.

This instrument is used to smooth off the edges of the nail in the nail groove. The file is gently placed in the nail groove against the free edge of the nail plate. The file is then gently pulled along the edge of the nail toward the end of the toe. This will smooth off any rough edges of the nail plate that may have been produced during the trimming or curetting procedures. This process may be repeated a number of times to make sure there are no rough edges remaining along the nail margin.

This file, like the curette, is mainly used along the nail margins of the great toenail. The lesser toenails do not usually require filing along their margins. By removing any sharp edges along the nail margin the possibility of the nail cutting into the soft tissues is reduced. As you become proficient in the use of this file you will find it to be an invaluable and time-saving instrument. Properly used it will add the professional finishing touch required in the care of toenails.

Properly used, a nail rasp will add the professional finishing touch to your nail service.

Diamond Nail File

To file the free edge of the toenails and in some cases to thin them, you may want to purchase a diamond nail file. Erica's Diamond Bits & Electric Files™[1] manufactures one type of file (Figure 8-4). It is metal with diamond dust impregnated in the metal. It comes in coarse, medium, and fine grits. For the toenails the coarse seems to work the best. It is constructed in such a manner that it does not fill up with nail debris during use. This file has the same shape as the nail files used by the nail professional for fingernail filing. It is thin and flexible and can be used in the same manner as other nail files. The major advantage of this file is that it is easily sanitized and can be kept in

---

[1] ATA Inc., Erica's Diamond Bits & Electric Files, 261 E. Broad St., Westerville, OH 43081, telephone 800-234-4717.

disinfectant solutions. It therefore can be used safely on many different clients. Because the file is metal and the cutting surface is made from diamond dust it is not easily worn out, making the initial expense extremely cost effective.

Foot File or Paddle

These are basically large sanding files made to remove dry flaky skin and smooth callus from the foot (Figure 8-5). They come in many different grits and shapes. Their main disadvantage is that they are not easily disinfected. Pick a file that can be sanitized and immersed in the disinfecting solution many times without falling apart. The Beautiful Feet™[2] foot file is well-constructed, easy to sanitize, and withstands the disinfectant solutions. It also lasts through many foot services, which makes it cost effective.

Creative Nail Design Systems™[3] supplies a foot paddle that has a disposable screen-like abrasive sanding surface. The paddle is easily taken apart so that the individual plastic parts can be sanitized and a new abrasive surface can be applied for the next client. The time spent and cost of reapplying abrasive is minimal, making this foot paddle cost effective with the added bonus of having a new abrasive surface for each client. Different abrasive grits may be applied to this file depending on the severity of the callus to be smoothed. This idea of a disposable cost-effective file is excellent and should be looked at closely by the nail professional.

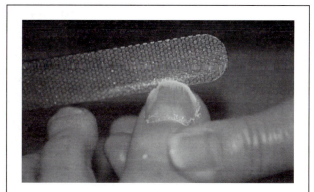

Figure 8-4 *The Erica's Diamond File™ being used on a toenail. This file can be kept in the disinfectant solution after it has been sanitized.*

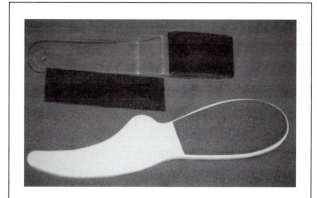

Figure 8-5 *Foot files by Creative Nail Design™ and Beautiful Feet™. They are easily sanitized and can be immersed in a disinfectant.*

Another alternative or addition to the foot file or paddle is a disposable pumice-like stone. Teregen Labs Pharmaceuticals™[4] manufactures such a product called the Pumbotti Pumi Bar. This product is designed to break down during its use so the tissue debris does not clog up the abrasive surface. It comes in three sizes and is a versatile product for removing dead skin from the feet. The small 1-inch size can be used once on individual clients very cost effectively.

---

[2] Beautiful Feet, 16632 Burke Ln, Huntington Beach, CA 92647, telephone 800-656-2646.

[3] Creative Nail Design Systems, 1125 Joshua Way, Vista, CA 92083, telephone 800-833-NAIL.

[4] Teregen Labs Pharmaceuticals, 38320 Western Parkway, Willoughby, OH 44095, telephone 800-848-0055.

The nail professional may want to have a combination of callus smoothing files. Each of these callus files has its advantages and disadvantages depending on the amount and type of callus that needs treatment. The cost is such that the nail professional could have three different files with different abrasive grits. This would allow the nail professional to easily tailor the service for the amount and type of callus to be smoothed.

All of these products may be sold to the client for home use. Clients must be cautioned and educated not to remove too much of the callus on their feet. To remove too much of this protective callus is not good for the underlying normal skin. Likewise when nail professionals smooth excess callus they must remove only enough to make the clients' skin smooth and comfortable. A thin layer of callus should remain to protect the underlying normal skin.

Callus removal requires care so that a thin layer of callus remains to protect the skin underneath.

Ingrown Nail Shaver

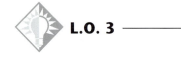

An ingrown nail shaver (see Figures 8-2 and 8-3) is optional but on occasion is a time saver when it comes to removing nail from along the nail groove of the big toenail. In most instances the small-angled nail rasp will be the instrument of choice for this job. Occasionally, however, a little more nail needs to be removed from the nail margin or a small "hook" or spicule of nail is present on the margin after trimming. The rasp would remove it but the shaver will do it safely and more quickly than the rasp. The instrument is shaped like a small paddle. There is a slot in the middle of the paddle and the end of the slot is filed to a sharp cutting edge. The paddle portion of the instrument is placed gently into the nail groove so that the edge of the nail edge is in the slot. If the nail edge does not slip easily into the slot then the nail rasp should be used to remove any unwanted portion of nail. Used gently and in the manner described this instrument can safely save time in trimming the nail margins of the great toe nail.

Cuticle Nippers

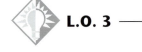

Little needs to be said about this instrument. The same instrument used for hand services can be used for foot services. It must be used carefully so as not to cut the living skin. On occasion you may use this instrument to remove a small portion of the nail corner in toes (two through five). Having smaller jaws than the nail nippers described previously, it is easier to use on the smaller toenails.

Drills

The electric drill is a time saver when working with thick, malformed toenails. Its use, however, is controversial within the nail industry. The main complaint about using the drill is that it is causing injury to a client's nails or to the soft tissues surrounding the nails. The answer to this is that the drill does not cause the injury! Improper use of the drill by an untrained operator causes these injuries, not the drill itself. With proper training and careful use, the drill becomes an extension of the user's fingers just as the other instruments used to perform nail services. Podiatrists may use the drill on almost every patient whose nails they trim. Without the electric drill their job would be much more complicated and time consuming.

Drills come in four basic types:

- Hand-held drill

- Cable-driven

- Belt-driven

- Micromotor

The secret of using any of these drills is to have a light touch and let the drill do the work. The hand-held type is basically made for wood-working and craft-making projects. The motor is incorporated into the handpiece. It has been adapted and used in the podiatry office as well as in nail salons for many years. For routine use on nail surfaces this type of drill may be awkward, unbalanced, and difficult to control.

Drills require a light touch. Improper use by a nail professional can injure the client.

The cable-driven drill has a handpiece attached to the motor by a cable encased within a flexible tube. This is an improvement over the hand-held type in that the handpiece is lighter, better balanced, and easier to control. Its disadvantages are that it must be hung, usually higher than the work area, so that the flexible tube and duplex spring in the handpiece remain relatively straight during use. If either of these are bent too much during use, the cable will kink or the duplex spring at the handpiece will break.

The belt- or cord-driven drill is basically the old type of drill used in dentistry. The handpiece is articulated on a metal arm attached to the motor. Power is transferred from the motor to the handpiece by a belt or cord that travels over pulleys mounted on the metal arm. The unit can be mounted on the wall by special mounts or on a weighted movable mount that can be set on the work table. A pedestal mount on wheels can be easily moved from one station to another. It is well balanced and easy to use. A disadvantage is that it needs more maintenance than the other two types of drills. The pulleys and handpiece must be oiled on a regular basis. The cord will have to be changed once in a while because it will wear out. One main advantage over the next type of drill we will discuss is that the electrical parts of this drill will be nowhere near the work area, which is generally wet when the foot service is given. This reduces the probability of electrical shock if the handpiece is accidently dropped into the water.

The micromotor drill is basically a miniaturized hand-held drill. The miniature motor is in the handpiece, which fits easily like a pencil in the hand. It is light, well balanced, and easily controlled. It requires minimal space in the work area. It is truly a professional instrument and its smooth vibration-free operation is appreciated by clients. This drill requires fairly low maintenance and is dependable. It is a bit more expensive than the other types; however, it will give many years of professional service, making it cost competitive with the other types of drills.

Drill Bits. These are the working parts of the drill. They come in many different shapes and are constructed of a number of different materials.

L.O. 5 A great deal of controversy and rhetoric within the professional nail industry involves what type of drill bits should be used for nail services. In this section we will try to give some insight on drill bits. Diamond or carbide? Coarse versus fine? What should you use? For foot services thinning the thick nail plate is the main purpose of drill use. Some special bits are made to smooth the rough skin and callus on the foot. The following discussion is about bits in general. Their use in providing foot services is discussed in Chapter 10.

Look at bits the same way you look at nail files—the coarser the file, the more it will cut. The finer files are made to polish. Basically drill bits are the same whether they be diamond or carbide. The coarser the cutting surface of the bit the faster it will cut or reduce the nail plate. The finer the cutting surface the slower it will cut the nail plate. Fine cutting surfaces polish more than they actually cut. Finer cutting surfaces also produce more heat than do coarser surfaces. Therefore, a lighter touch must be used when using a fine cutting or polishing bit. If used improperly any of these bits will injure the soft tissues underlying and around the nail.

Which bits should you use? It all depends on what you wish to do to the nail. If the nail needs thinning, a pear-shaped coarse cutting bit is the best. Used with a light touch you can remove nail polish without cutting into the nail plate. If you wish to remove nail thickness slightly more pressure is applied. Excess nail is quickly removed in this manner. The main thing to remember is to keep the bit moving quickly over the surface of the nail plate so heat does not build up. Certain diamond bits will also work for this purpose. If smoothing and polishing the nail is necessary a fine diamond bit may be used. Purchase good quality bits whether they be diamond or carbide. The ultimate is to find a bit that can be used for most of your nail work and then practice with it. Try to use one bit for the major part of your work. You may need one or two others on occasion for special circumstances. Changing bits for each different process is time consuming and unnecessary.

Choice of drill bit depends on the job to be done.

EQUIPMENT

In this section we discuss the various large equipment items necessary to provide a pedicure service. These can be as simple as a folding chair and a plastic dish pan to the elegant, fully-plumbed pedicure unit. Quality equipment will be cost effective and also will help to promote your foot services. When purchasing this equipment think of yourself as well as your clients. Purchase equipment that makes it as comfortable and as easy as possible for you to provide the service. If you are uncomfortable and awkward in the provision of the service, this feeling will be transferred to your clients. When you are relaxed your client can then relax and enjoy the pedicure. You will not be inclined to promote or provide foot services if they are not comfortable and easy for you.

Clients know what they want and in many cases believe that expensive professional equipment indicates a better quality of service. No matter what equipment you purchase make sure that it appears professional and is comfortable. Purchase within your budget but do not cut corners. Try not to purchase the same type of equipment that the client can purchase for home use. If you do, clients will be wondering why they are paying to soak their feet in your salon instead of doing it for free at home. For this reason, purchase only quality professional equipment and you will be money and clients ahead. Let us discuss equipment that in general is not for home use.

Pedicure Carts

These units are basically a stool on wheels. The pedicurist straddles and sits on the cart. This position can be awkward and uncomfortable. There are many different designs and manufacturers of these carts. Be sure the height of the cart is such that you will look down on the foot. This will tend to keep your back straighter and you will be more relaxed when giving the service. There is usually a built-in footrest for the client's feet. There are also drawers and shelves for storage of instruments and pedicure materials (Figure 8-6). Some of these units even include a space for the foot bath on the front of the cart. The units are compact and take up little space in the salon. They are also inexpensive. For the salon that has only limited space for pedicure services the pedicure cart is the unit of choice. If space is available for upgrading the pedicure area, then consider a more professional arrangement.

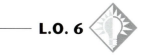
L.O. 6

Be sure the equipment you purchase is comfortable for you and your clients.

Water Baths

These come as simple as a plastic pan to a fully-plumbed self-contained hydrotherapy spa. Your budget will determine what you use. In making your choice think like a client. If you were receiving the pedicure, what would you

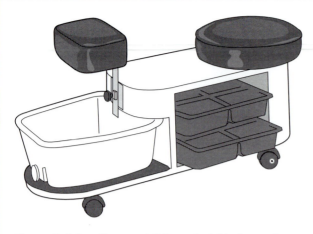

Figure 8-6 *A pedicure cart. It is comfortable, has a place for the foot bath, a storage area for supplies, and an adjustable foot rest.*

A whirlpool foot spa is the ultimate luxury for your clients.

like your feet soaked in? Go for it in this purchase! Your clients' first impression of their pedicure starts here. A dime store plastic tub is not the purchase to make.

Small portable water baths with vibrators and heaters built into the them are available. These are a step above the plastic pan and combined with the full service of the pedicure are satisfactory. The main problem is they must be manually filled and emptied after each client service. Also clients can purchase this type of water bath for themselves. Because of this, they are not the special treat that the client is paying for in the pedicure. If you use the portable type be sure to have a special comfortable chair or lounge in a private or semiprivate area for the client to sit in while receiving the pedicure. The chair should be on a platform to save your back during the service.

A step above the portable water bath is the custom-built pedicure units that have a removable foot bath built into the unit (Figure 8-7). These are constructed with both the client and the nail professional in mind. They add elegance to the service and make it much easier for the nail professional

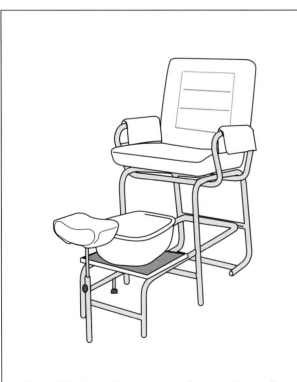

Figure 8-7 *A semi-throne type pedicure station, well-built, and affordable. It has an adjustable foot rest and a place for the water bath.*

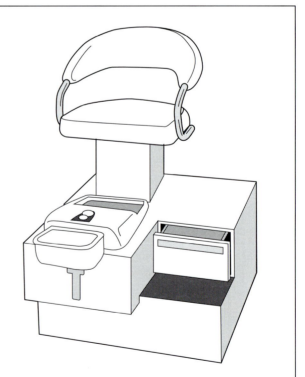

Figure 8-8 *A pedicare center is well constructed with a removable foot bath, storage drawer, and adjustable foot rest.*

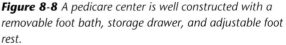

to perform the pedicure. One company that builds such a unit is Pibbs Industries.[5] Their pedicure unit is a pedestal design with a removable water bath (like in Figure 8-8). It is moderately priced and well accepted by clients. They also have another very basic designed pedestal unit at about half the price, which is also quite serviceable.

Portable foot spas have built-in whirlpools and can be filled from the sink. After the service they drain the water by pumping the water back into the sink drain. They have built-in footrests and areas for storage of the pedicure materials. They add an extra elegance to the service by the gentle massaging action of the whirlpool. European Touch Ltd. II[6] has a unit like this (similar to Figure 8-9). This unit may also be purchased with both a client chair and the pedicurist's chair. These have been specifically designed to comple-ment the portable foot spa. The cost of the unit is slightly higher than the custom-built unit but you may find the added benefit of the whirlpool and self-draining features well worth the expense.

The ultimate pedicure foot bath is the fully-plumbed pedicure spa chair. European Touch Ltd. II produces a deluxe well-designed unit (like Figure 8-10). This unit is not portable and must be planned for when design-ing the pedicure area of your salon. It is attached to both hot and cold water as well as to a drain. If a floor drain is not available a pump option may be purchased, which will pump the water to an available drain. The unit also has a built-in massage feature in the client chair, which adds to the relaxation of the pedi-cure. It is easily sanitized and disinfected. The $3000 price range may seem high, but if you consider client satisfaction and referral potential the initial expense may be well worth it. This type of unit will last a long while and during that peri-od will pay for itself many times over. Other com-panies manufacture fully-plumbed less expensive units.

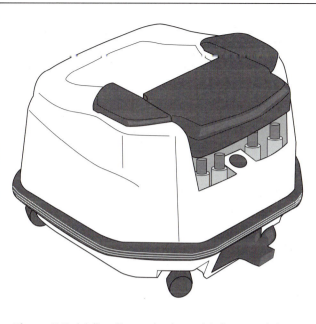

Figure 8-9 A fully self-contained portable foot spa. It is a step above the previously discussed pedicure furnishings.

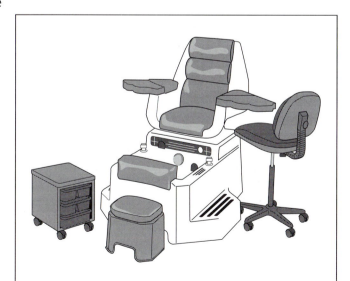

Figure 8-10 A elite, fully-plumbed, throne type, pedicure unit. It comes with many options including a massage unit built into the client chair which the client can control.

[5] Pibbs® Industries, 133-15 32nd Ave., Flushing, NY 11354, telephone 800-551-5020, FAX 718-461-3910.
[6] European Touch Ltd. II, P.O. Box 322, Brookfield, WI 53008-0322, telephone 800-626-6912.

No matter which water bath unit you purchase be sure to purchase a seat for yourself that fits both you and the unit. Sit on a number of stools or chairs supplied with the units and see if they are uncomfortable or inefficient when it comes to actually providing the service. Also, are they too short to allow the legs to be placed in a comfortable position? It seems **ergonomic** design, which maximizes productivity by minimizing operator fatigue and discomfort, has not as yet been incorporated into the pedicurist's seat. If at all possible look for a stool or chair that is adjustable for height. Your back will love you for it!

FOOT NOTES

This chapter has discussed the basic instruments and equipment necessary in the provision of professional pedicures. Too many nail professionals in the industry are being penny wise and dollar poor when it comes to purchasing instruments and equipment. If you get one thing out of this chapter it must be that quality professional tools and equipment are the cost-effective purchases for you to make. Cheap, modified instruments and equipment wear out faster and make your job harder to perform. The result, if one wishes to provide a quality service, is continual replacement of these items. Do not save pennies when it will cost you dollars over the life of your practice. Shop for price but do not sacrifice quality! Professional quality should always be your "buy" word!

QUESTIONS

1. Why is the pumice stone not recommended for pedicuring use in the salon?

2. What are the five basic instruments recommended for a foot care service?

3. Why should toenails be trimmed using the nail nippers like a pair of scissors instead of trying to trim the entire nail in one cut?

4. What are the four basic types of electric drills? Do electric drills injure clients?

5. Why is it preferable to use a coarse drill bit when grinding down a thick toenail?

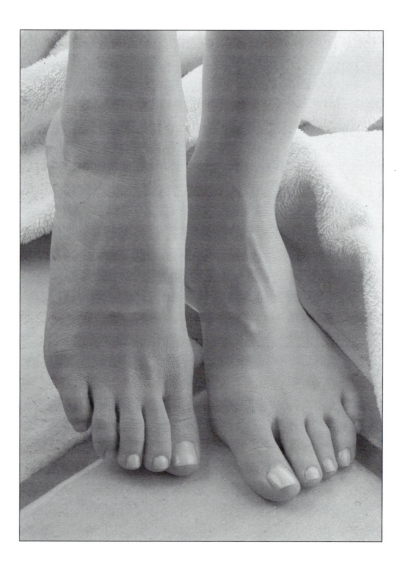

Sanitation in the Workplace | 9

LEARNING OBJECTIVES

After studying this chapter, the reader should be able to:

1. Explain the importance of good housekeeping and the client's first impression.

2. Define sanitation, disinfection, and sterilization.

3. Briefly discuss the early attempts at disinfection in medicine.

4. Define normal flora and cite examples.

5. Describe the typical pathogenic organisms found in a salon.

6. Describe the five categories of biocidal agents.

7. Explain the advantages and disadvantages of the various disinfectant classes.

8. Discuss the factors that can affect the action of disinfectants.

9. Explain and interpret a label on a disinfectant container.

10. Describe a well-designed and furnished salon.

The place in which you work is a reflection of you. Your clients' first impressions of you will be formed by the area or place in which you perform your services. It has been said repeatedly, "you have only one chance to make a first impression." Considering this you had better make the most of it! This chapter will discuss your workplace, particularly the pedicure area, and the important points that you must observe to keep a happy, contented, healthy clientele who will refer you new clients. You can be the best, most qualified nail professional in your area but if the public does not perceive this you will not be successful.

S A L O N   S A N I T A T I O N

Sanitation practices MUST begin at the front door of your salon!

One might wonder why this subject is covered in a chapter on the workplace. It is because sanitation practices must start at the front door of the salon and be implemented in every area of the workplace. If you were to visit your doctor and noticed a dirty reception room would you not start wondering about the cleanliness of the rest of the office? Your salon is perceived by your clients in the same way as they do their doctors' offices. You are giving a personal service just as a doctor does. You touch your clients just as a doctor touches patients. You use instruments on clients just as a doctor uses instruments on patients. Your salon must therefore be as sanitary as your doctor's office. The public today demands this! Many patients may believe they got an infection from the unsanitary practices of their pedicurist. In most instances this is not true but there is nothing you can say that will change their belief. In some way their pedicurist failed to impart to clients that they were being served in a professional manner within a sanitary, disease-free environment. Because of the dark moist environment created by hosiery and shoes, the foot is an excellent candidate for infections of many kinds. Sanitation practices must be scrupulously observed by those who provide foot services. Clients will be much more understanding if they believe their pedicurist has tried to prevent infections by giving professional service in a clean, disinfected surrounding.

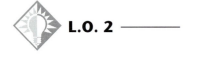

L.O. 1

A clean, orderly, well kept salon must be the first impression a client has of your place of business. This is the beginning step in salon sanitation—it is basically housekeeping. Dusting the furniture, sweeping or vacuuming the floors, cleaning the rest room and maintaining a clean, uncluttered work area will go a long way toward keeping a satisfied client. Once your clients realize that they are being served in a clean workplace it will then be easy for you to talk to them about the disinfection methods you use within your salon for their protection.

Within the beauty industry we are seeing the interchange of the terms sanitize and disinfect. These are two different terms and are not interchangeable. The medical dictionary defines these terms as follows:

L.O. 2

◆ **Sanitization**—to clean, as one would eating or drinking utensils. This word is derived from the word sanitary, which is defined as promoting or pertaining to health.

◆ **Disinfection**—to free from pathogenic organisms or to render them inert.

These two terms are not the same and should not be interchanged. By maintaining a clean workplace one is promoting health. The cleaning or sanitization of the workplace is in reality reducing the probability of the transmission of disease within that area to an acceptable level. In another sense this process allows you to work and your clients to be served in a healthy environment.

The next higher level of the process is disinfection. This process must always be preceded by sanitizing, or cleaning, the surfaces to be disinfected. This means washing your hands, instruments, and work surfaces to remove organic and inorganic matter before the disinfection process is started. *Washing is the most important part of the whole procedure.* The disinfection process is used on surfaces or objects that come into contact with the client and the beauty professional within the salon. This includes all work surfaces, all tools and instruments including files and drills, and last, but by far from least, the hands, including yours as well as your client's. In the process of disinfection the majority of the disease-causing (**pathogenic**) organisms are destroyed or rendered inert. This is the subtle but important difference between these two terms. In sanitization we are not necessarily destroying organisms but only reducing their numbers to acceptable levels. In disinfection the disease-causing organisms or pathogens are actually destroyed or at least rendered inert or incapable of producing disease.

For completeness of this section the term sterilization needs to be discussed.

◆ **Sterilization**—process which completely eliminates all microbial **viability** (life).

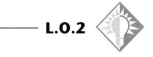 L.O.2

The most important practice to prevent the spread of infection is WASHING—your hands, your instruments, and the work surfaces.

Generally sterilization is not necessary in the salon setting. Because of the nature of their services, estheticians are required to sterilize certain instruments but for other beauty and nail professionals the process is not necessary. The use of proper disinfecting procedures and products will reduce the number of pathogenic organisms to acceptable levels within the general salon setting.

Early Events that Lead to the Disinfecting Process

Disease and disease-causing organisms have been present since the beginning of time. It is only in the last 200 years that we have been able to connect specific bacteria or other microscopic organisms to the diseases they produce. The Egyptians had a vague notion that certain diseases could be transmitted by touch. Many societies before the birth of Christ felt that disease was of Divine origin. Hippocrates rejected this theory but had no idea that microorganisms were involved in the disease process. In 1546, Fracastorius was the first to propose a germ theory for disease. In 1609, Galileo and Jansen independently invented the compound telescope. Anthony van Leeuwenhoek in

1676 modified the telescope to a microscope, which enabled him to actually observe and identify individual microorganisms. In the Dark Ages there was little advancement in the study of microorganisms. In 1860 Pasteur developed the **pasteurization** process and in so doing proved that microorganisms actually produced disease. Shortly thereafter, Joseph Lister applied **carbolic acid (phenol)**-soaked dressings to surgical wounds thus reducing infections after surgery. About the same time others in Germany and France used bleach for the same purpose. The idea of washing the hands in these same solutions before surgery followed next. Thus, the beginnings of sanitization and disinfection practices arose. Today we still practice many of the basic principles of disinfection developed by these early pioneers.

L.O. 3

Microbial Organisms Commonly Present in the Salon

L.O. 4

Normal flora. Our bodies are covered with bacteria and other organisms that we cannot see. They are a normal inhabitant, called normal **flora**, and until they are allowed to overgrow or to penetrate the skin or mucous membranes they will not cause disease. Most of the normal flora found on our skin are not permanent residents but transferred from other areas of the body or from the environment by our hands or other objects.

Some examples of normal flora are:

1. Staphylococcus epidermidis—a bacteria

2. Streptococcus—a bacteria

3. Various fungi

Under normal circumstances organisms will not cause disease or infection in humans.

Under normal circumstances these organisms will not cause disease or infection in humans. However, with a portal of entry (a cut or abrasion) they can then cause a disease process to arise. Proper sanitization and disinfection techniques will lower the probabilities of an infection should the beauty professional inadvertently cause a portal of entry.

Some people have normal flora that under the same conditions on another person would cause an infection or disease. These people are called **carriers**. These pathogenic organisms that they normally carry do not produce disease within that person. They may be transferred to others where they will produce disease. Proper disinfection technique and procedures will protect you as well as your clients from an individual who is a carrier. Some people will show evidence of actual disease (fungal or bacterial infections) that can be spread to others unless proper precautions are taken. Knowing what precautions to take and how to take them is that much more important under these circumstances.

There are literally billions of organisms in the environment but not all cause disease. Certain of these organisms are more prevalent in particular environments. In the confined space of the salon, because of the services provided and the numbers of clients served, organisms are concentrated and therefore found in greater numbers. Typical pathogenic organisms occurring in large concentrations within a salon are fungi, yeast, molds, bacteria, and viruses.

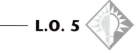 L.O. 5

Fungi. The **dermatophyte** classes grow on glabrous skin (smooth or bare), scalp, hair, or nails. These can be transmitted from client to client at areas of recently abraded skin, hair, or nails.

Yeast (candida). Yeast cause superficial infections of mucous membranes and areas of the skin that stay warm and moist such as between the toes and along nail folds.

Molds. These are actually another form of fungi that grow in dry areas such as the nails. They are for the most part dry and dust-like in their growth (i.e., penicillin mold on bread).

Fungi, molds, and yeasts all form spores. A spore is a single cell with a hard outer coating like an egg. Spores therefore are extremely resistant to physical and environmental changes. A spore under the right condition can cause infection. Spores are difficult to destroy. Even some bacteria can form spores.

We are fortunate that the billions of organisms in the environment don't all cause disease.

Bacteria. Bacteria, both pathogenic and nonpathogenic, are everywhere. However, in enclosed public places bacteria are much more concentrated. Salon professionals must be aware of this and have good protocols in place to sanitize the salon and disinfect surfaces that come into contact with themselves and their clients. A **bactericidal disinfectant** is a necessity.

Virus. Viruses—influenza, **adenovirus**, **vaccinia**, herpes simplex, HIV, and **hepatitis** types A and B—are all found in places where people congregate and thus are found also in the salon. An ideal disinfectant for the salon should also be viru**cidal**. Today everyone is worried about HIV. Hepatitis type B is more easily transmitted from one person to another than HIV. More doctors and health care workers are infected with type B hepatitis than HIV. This virus can be transmitted by contact with blood, blood serum, saliva, or other body fluids. Although at the present we have no vaccine against HIV, there is one available for type B hepatitis. For this reason all health care workers are now offered the vaccine and in some cases are required to take it before employment. Beauty professionals because of their close contact with clients should seriously consider obtaining this vaccination. Some insurance companies are now covering this vaccine, which makes it more available to the general population. Check with your doctor.

Five Categories of Disinfectants or Biocidal Agents

Biocidal agents are those that destroy living organisms. The five categories are:

L.O. 6

1. **Iodophors**—These are disinfectants in which the active ingredient is iodine. They act on the organisms by separating and breaking down the cellular proteins.

2. **Alcohols**—The active ingredient in these disinfectants is usually isopropyl alcohol. There can be others such as ethyl, methyl, or benzyl alcohols. These act by **denaturation** of proteins (splitting of the molecular structure), interference with metabolism, or actual **lysis** (dissolving) of the organism.

3. **Phenolics**—The active ingredient here is phenol also known as **Carbolic acid**. Phenol is an extremely poisonous compound so for use as a disinfectant must be diluted. Phenolics act as disinfectants by disruption of the cell wall, **precipitation** of proteins, inactivation of **enzymes**, and as cytoplasmic (fluid within the cell surrounding the nucleus) poisons. Phenol in itself is so bactericidal that other disinfectants are measured against its bactericidal activity to determine their own strength in killing bacteria. This is called the **"phenol coefficient."**

4. **Quaternary ammonium compounds (QUATS)**—The available ammonium or chloride portions of these disinfectants are the active ingredients. They act by denaturation of proteins, inactivation of cellular metabolites, and dissolution of the cell wall.

5. **Glutaraldehydes**—The aldehyde portion of these disinfectants is the active ingredient. They are a general poison. WARNING: Extreme care must be taken when using this product. Even inhaling small quantities of this disinfectant can cause injury to the user. Hospitals are now requiring employees who work around this material to wear a dose badge that will tell how much vapor has been inhaled.

Advantages and Disadvantages of the Five Classes of Disinfectants

L.O. 7

Before choosing a disinfectant the user must weigh the various advantages and disadvantages of each class. Only in so doing will one arrive at an optimal product for use in the individual salon. First review Table 9-1 that lists the various advantages and disadvantages of each class.

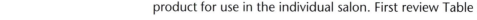

Advantages and Disadvantages of Various Disinfectants

DISINFECTANT	ADVANTAGE	DISADVANTAGE
Alcohols	Easily obtainable, tuberculocidal, bacteriocidal, in most instances will not harm work surfaces	Not good cleaning agents, easily weakened by organic matter, flammable, corrosive to metal
Iodophors	Are effective against some viruses, act quickly to destroy organisms, are effective against **gram-positive** and some **gram-negative** bacteria	Not good for cleaning, may stain surfaces, are inactivated by heat and ultraviolet light, weakened by organic materials, water will decrease activity
QUATS	Excellent against gram-positive bacteria, inhibit bacterial growth in high concentrations, fairly stable in water, are nonstaining, may be used on work surfaces	Can cause staining on materials, not effective against certain viruses, minimally active against fungus, generally not tuberculocidal, affected by hard water, organic material decreases activity
Phenolics	Have broad spectrum biocidal activity, generally **fungicidal** as well as tuberculocidal, can work in presence of organic matter, have been used for a long while	Have a hospital odor, can cause rubber and plastics to swell, some organic materials reduce activity, some communities impose disposal restrictions, may cause brownish discoloration of nails
Glutaraldehydes	Only class that is **sporocidal**, under proper conditions can be used as a sterilizer, tuberculocidal and **virucidal**, in some formulations have long shelf life, in most instances are nonstaining and relatively noncorrosive to metals	Will irritate mucous membranes, are toxic if inhaled at more than .5 parts per million, can cause skin irritations, unstable in solution, heavy organic matter inactivates them, must be in an alkaline or basic solution to maintain activity, will damage work surfaces

Table 9-1

Factors Affecting the Action of Disinfectants

Many factors cause the action of disinfectants to be enhanced or reduced. Taking these factors into consideration, along with the advantages and disadvantages, will enable the user to select the proper disinfectant for the proper job.

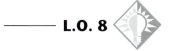

The Dilution of the Disinfectant. Many of the disinfectants come to the user as a concentrated product and must be diluted before use. WARNING: It is important to follow the manufacturer's recommendations in mixing the product for use. Too little and the product will not be strong enough and conversely too much will in most cases reduce the strength. The optimum action of the individual disinfectants will be at its own specific dilution.

Dwell Time. The amount of time the disinfectant is in contact with the organism is often called dwell time. The longer the disinfectant is in contact with the organism the greater the probability of its destroying that organism. This has a down side in that the disinfectant in many cases will damage the surface on which the organism is living if it is left in contact with it for too long a period. There is therefore an optimum dwell time for each disinfectant depending on the surface being disinfected. Follow the manufacturer's instructions!

Diluent. The diluent or solution in which the concentrate is mixed (e.g., whether your water is hard or soft) will determine to a great extent how effective your disinfectant will be. A high percentage of minerals in the water (hard water) will decrease the effectiveness of the disinfectant. To determine how hard your local water supply is contact your water or utilities company. If the hardness is over 60 parts per million you should use distilled or bottled water to mix your disinfectants.

Soil Contaminants. This refers to the type of contaminant on the surface you wish to disinfect. Contaminants can be blood, grease, hair, urine, dirt, soap, residue, and so forth. Organic or inorganic matter, in even small amounts, can inactivate most disinfectants. It is important that you sanitize or clean the surfaces to be disinfected before you actually disinfect them! Also if you observe nail filings or other debris in your disinfecting tray you must realize the disinfectant activity of the solution has been decreased. Change the solution whenever you observe debris in it and also as often as recommended by the manufacturer. This is a very important part of the disinfecting process.

pH. The pH refers to whether something is acidic or basic in nature. Lemons are acidic; baking soda and antacids such as Mylanta™ are basic. The pH scale is a scale from 1 to 14. Seven is a neutral pH; from 1 to 6.9 is acidic, and from 7.1 to 14 is basic. Organisms live between pH 3.5 to 9.5. Therefore, if the disinfectant pH is within this range it will not destroy all the organisms, that is, if the pH is 4, organisms between 4.5 to 9.5 will not be affected. Conversely, if the pH is between 0 and 2 or between 11 and 14, the acid or base will act on the surface you are trying to disinfect or yourself in a detrimental manner (Figure 9-1). What pH is then best for disinfection? On the acid side of the scale it is between 2.6 and 3.2 and on the basic side it is between 10 and 11. In these areas harm to the environmental surfaces is minimized while microbial destruction is enhanced. Contact or dwell time is critical! Too much time will cause damage to the surfaces being disinfected and not enough time will not allow for proper disinfection to occur.

Temperature. Temperature can affect the activity of the disinfectant. Too high or too low a temperature can decrease the killing power or activity of the disinfectant. Follow the manufacturer's recommendations on this matter.

You are the most important factor in the entire disinfection process! If you do not choose the right materials, if you do not follow the manufacturer's recommendations, or if you do not develop and follow proper disinfection procedures for your salon or work area, all your efforts will be for naught.

YOU are the most important factor in maintaining a clean environment for your clients.

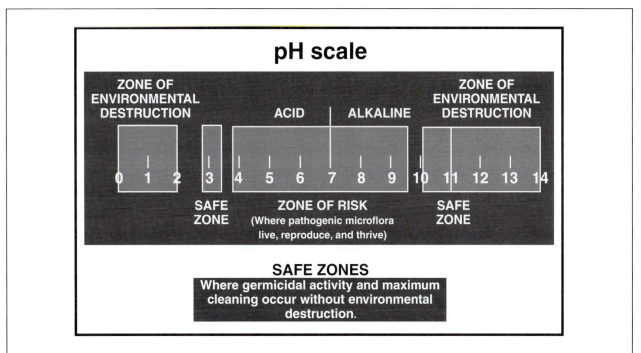

Figure 9-1 *Diagram of the pH scale shows the range where the disinfection process is optimum. These are called the safe zones on the scale. If the disinfectant pH falls within these ranges pathogenic microorganisms are destroyed or rendered inert in the optimum dwell time with minimum harm being done to other environmental surfaces or organisms.*

What Does the Label Mean?

The labels of the various products tell what the active ingredient in the product is as well as what organisms it will effectively destroy or render inert. To make these claims on the label the product must undergo rigorous testing against specific organisms. These tests are performed under the direction of the Association of Analytical Chemists. After passing the tests the product is then registered with the U.S. Environmental Protection Agency (EPA) and given an EPA registration number. This number must be displayed on the label. If you do not find an EPA registration number on the product, the product is not for use as a disinfectant in the salon. Table 9-2 lists claims found on labels and the organisms that must be tested against before the claim can be listed on the label.

—— **L.O. 9**

How to Select Disinfectants for the Salon

To select the proper disinfectant one must first determine the level of antimicrobial activity necessary for the specific conditions in which it will be used. You then decide how the various advantages and disadvantages can be balanced to give the best job under those specific conditions. What this basically says is that you cannot use a single class of disinfectants for everything, that is, cleaning work surfaces, instruments, walls, bathrooms, or your hands. You would not use the same disinfectant to wash your hands as you would use to disinfect work surfaces or your instruments.

LABEL	ORGANISM	NOTES
Germicide/ Disinfectant	*Salmonella choleraesuis*	Must be able to destroy gram-negative organisms
General purpose/ Broad spectrum	*Staphylococcus aureus, Salmonella choleraesuis,* and one other organism of manufacturer's choice	
Hospital disinfectant	*Salmonella choleraesuis, Staphylococcus aureus,* and two other bacterial organisms of manufacturer's choice	
Fungicidal	*Trichophyton mentagrophytes*	Other fungi can and should be tested for, particularly *Trichophyton rubrum,* which is prevalent and more resistant than *Trichophyton mentagrophytes,* however this is not a requirement
Tuberculocidal	*Mycobacterium tuberculosis*	To destroy tuberculosis means it is strong enough to provide better overall coverage for other organisms, but these products are strong enough to harm the surfaces being disinfected—questionable for salon use
Virucidal	Lipophilic viruses	These are viruses that combine with or dissolve in fats
Sporocidal	*Bacillus subtilis, Clostridium sporogenes*	These products also may be called a sterilizing agent only if it has passed all the other tests

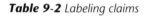

Table 9-2 *Labeling claims*

Read and understand product labels. The following is a typical label found on a disinfectant sold at the various trade shows. Let us look at it rather critically.

Typical Label

◆ Highly effective dual quaternary disinfectant

◆ Disinfectant + Cleaner + Germicide + Fungicidal + Virucide + Sanitizer + Deodorizer

◆ Effective against 63 pathogens including: HIV-1, Herpes 1 and 2, Polio, Measles, Salmonella, and Influenza

---

The first thing we notice on this label is that it is a QUATS. From this we know what category of disinfectant it is and can begin comparing the advantages and disadvantages of the product. By doing this it can be determined whether the product is compatible with what is to be disinfected (bathrooms, work surfaces, instruments, floors, etc.). The next thing this label tells us is that it is a disinfectant. If you will notice it actually says this twice and without knowing anything else about the product we know that it is at least a toilet bowl cleaner that has been tested against *Salmonella choleraesuis*. Reading further it informs us it is also a cleaner so it can be used to wash things. Next it tells us it is a germicide, which we already know because it has previously stated that it is a disinfectant. The label finally becomes more informative when it states that it is a fungicide as well as a virucide. This tells us it has been tested against *Trichophyton mentagrophytes* fungus and lipophilic virus. The next thing it tells us is that it is a sanitizer as well as a deodorizer. Literally it tells us it "promotes health" and while doing so it also deodorizes.

The last part of the label states it is effective against 63 pathogenic organisms including the certain ones listed. The question to ask the dealer is what 63 organisms is the product effective against? One would think it had not been tested against *Staphylococcus aureus*, otherwise the label would have stated it was a broad-spectrum disinfectant. Also has it been tested against *Pseudomonas aeruginosa*? If so, it should have been labeled a hospital disinfectant. As you can see labels are important in what they tell us about the product. More importantly one should be more aware of what the label does not say!

This product is satisfactory for use in the salon. It basically is effective against most of the organisms found in the salon setting. It may be used on work surfaces as well as instruments. The main problem with this product is the labeling. If we looked at the 63 pathogens it is effective against we would find that it had been tested against the proper organisms. There is another disinfectant being sold to the nail professional with identical active ingredients. This product has more specific labeling, which would make it more satisfactory for use except it comes premixed, which makes it very expensive for use in the salon.

Cleaning and disinfecting will eventually be second nature to you. It just takes practice!

What Next?

Once products for cleaning and disinfecting the salon have been chosen it is up to you to make them work properly. This is not a complicated or time-consuming process. Once you have practiced basic disinfecting techniques in the salon, the process becomes second nature. You will do it because it is the way things are done in your workplace for the protection of yourself as well as your clients. Be aware of the factors affecting the action of disinfectants and make them work for you. This is done by following the manufacturer's instructions exactly. For instance, if the product is a concentrate it will need to be mixed in the proper proportions to ensure optimum action of the disinfectant. The containers the solutions are kept in must be cleaned each time the solutions are changed. Change the solutions at the intervals recommended by the manufacturer or whenever foreign organic material or other debris is observed in them. Sanitize all instruments, drill bits, and other tools before placing them in the disinfectant solutions. Make sure the objects to be disinfected are in contact with the disinfectant for the prescribed period of time recommended by the manufacturer.

FOOT NOTES

You are the most important part of the disinfection process! It is your responsibility to develop procedures for disinfection practices in your salon. You must choose products that will work adequately within the different areas of the salon. You must understand how they work and see that they are used properly. You must be an educated consumer. Educate your clients about your salon sanitation practices so they understand they are being served in a healthy, disease-free environment. They will appreciate your concern for their well-being and refer others to you because of it.

Educate your clients about your salon sanitation practices so they understand they are being served in a healthy, disease-free environment.

Never forget that basic hygiene practices, like washing your hands between clients, are the beginning of the disinfecting process. The use of topical gel disinfectants for the hands does not take the place of basic washing. The skin oils, dead skin, and nail dust all are organic compounds and will decrease the effectiveness of these products. Washing your hands as well as those of your client with soap and water is important. Application of the topical disinfectants after washing will then reduce microorganisms to much lower acceptable levels on the hands. Nothing will take the place of the basic hand-washing practice! Use only instruments and tools that may be washed and disinfected between clients. Always change disinfectant solutions if any foreign material is observed in the solution and at least as often as recommended by the manufacturer.

AREAS OF THE SALON

As in a doctor's office or any other place of service, the first impression con-
sumers have of that doctor or business is the waiting room and the reception ——— L.O. 10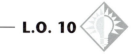
person who receives them. No expense should be held back in making this
area an inviting place that demonstrates to clients you care about their comfort. This area must be clean, bright, and relaxing. It should be large enough
so the clients will not feel crowded. Comfortable chairs make for a home-like
atmosphere and give each client individual space. Have you ever noticed in a
waiting room that the individual chairs will be used before a couch or lounge?
Humans, particularly strangers, each need their own comfortable space before
they can relax and begin to interact with others. Decorate the walls with pictures you like. Generally your clients will like them also and compliment you
on them. Keep a good selection of up to date magazines for your clients'
enjoyment. A well-designed brochure outlining your services should also be
available in this area. The reception area should not be directly open to the
service areas of your salon. You or the client you are working on should not
be distracted by the conversations or business that occurs in the reception
area. Take a few moments to sit in your reception area before or after work. If
you find it relaxing so will your clients.

Clients do not enjoy reading magazines that are months, or even years, old. Keep your reading materials up to date!

As clients move from the reception area into the working areas of the
salon they should continue to observe a clean, well-kept setting. The work
stations where nail services are rendered should be uncluttered and sanitary.
Instruments and tools should be in the proper disinfectant solutions that are
free of any organic debris. There *must* be a sink area where the nail professional as well as the clients wash their hands. Ideally there should be a sink for
every two or three stations. This area can also be used to wash used instruments and tools between client services before they are placed back into the
disinfectant solutions. Too many nail professionals work in salons that do not
have a sink within the salon. It is down the hall or in another area of the complex, or at the least it is inaccessible and inconvenient for them to use. This is
unacceptable for a personal service place of business. If you work in such a
place you must demand an accessible sink for sanitation practices and if it is
not furnished find another salon to work in that does have sinks. If you do not
your clients surely will!

The sink area of the salon is an excellent place to also display the
products you use when servicing your clients. While standing there washing
their hands what more do they have to do than look at these products. For
people to become interested in a product they have to be reminded of it at
least three times. In your salon the reception room display is the first, the sink
display may be the second, and the third is when you are actually using the

various products on the client. The client will begin to ask questions and it is then easy to educate the client about the products and what benefits they have. This becomes even more important in the foot service areas because many products will be of great benefit to a client's foot health.

The lighting in the salon should be first class. A well-lighted area creates a sense of well-being. It also reduces eye strain on the nail professional. Extra work lights at the work stations are a requirement and the ones with a built-in magnifier are helpful when working along the nail margins of toenails. Mood lighting in the foot service areas is a great client relaxer. Proper use of track lighting and dimmer switches will help to make the pedicure service one the client will want to repeat.

Relaxing background music will benefit you and your clients.

A sound system for music will go a long way to relax your clients as well as yourself. One suggestion is a system with built-in speakers and its own tuner amplifier. A compact disk (CD) player addition will allow you to control the type of music being played much more easily than a radio. The music being played should be as soothing and nondistracting as possible. Try different types of music from country to classical to new age. Then decide on a type appropriate for you and your clients. Nail and foot services should be provided in the most relaxed environment possible.

The foot service areas should be separate from the other areas of the salon. Most people think their feet are ugly or they are self-conscious about showing their feet to others. Receiving the foot service in a private surrounding will solve these problems. It also promotes relaxation, which should be one of the main benefits of a professionally provided foot service. These private areas may each be decorated in a different theme. For instance an ocean room could be decorated with pictures of ocean scenes, maritime memorabilia, fish, and so forth. Your clients will look forward to trying different theme rooms for their pedicures depending on how they feel that day. Mood lighting and personal earphones with relaxation tapes of ocean sounds and music all will make the foot service more enjoyable and an experience the client will want to repeat. The possibilities are limited only by your imagination.

Set up each room or area so that it is comfortable for you to work. A work table for your instruments and equipment begins the setup. The work table may be portable or stationary. It should be at the proper height for easy use and large enough so that it appears uncluttered during the service. There should be an instrument container for your disinfectant solution and instruments. There must also be an instrument tray on which to place the instruments you will be using for that particular service. Do not lay the instruments on the work surface before or after use. Clients will look at this practice as being unsanitary. If you use a drill it should be easily accessible either on top of the work area or hanging from the side. Lotions, massage oils, and other materials used for the pedicure should have their own particular place on or in the table. Drawers may contain these items and also hold towels or any other materials necessary for the pedicure. If you are right-handed the table should be placed on your right, and on the left, if you are left-handed.

Take time to pick a comfortable chair, stool, or pedicure cart on which you will sit. This should be on wheels so you can move easily into the various positions necessary to provide the service. It must be the proper height for you to be comfortable during the provision of the service. A covered waste container should be easily accessible. If the work table is custom designed this container may be built into it. A chair for clients to sit on while removing their footgear is also necessary. This may be the same chair they sit in while receiving the service, however, if a custom pedestal type setup is used for the pedicure another chair in the area for dressing purposes is desirable. A special shelf or stand next to the dressing chair for the footgear to be placed on gives an added touch of thought and professionalism.

Sanitation in the pedicure areas must be scrupulous. Your clients will demand it. Make sure that the foot baths and surrounding areas are sanitized and disinfected between each client. Remember the difference between sanitize and disinfect? You will sanitize the floors and chairs. You will sanitize and disinfect the actual work surfaces that come into contact with you and the client. This includes areas such as the water bath and footrest as well as your instruments. A sink for this purpose *must* be available within the salon.

How the client is placed for the service will depend on the type of foot bath you decide on for your pedicure service. For your comfort, the client chair should be placed on a raised platform. Some custom designed moderately priced pedicure chairs and the fully-plumbed spa chairs come with the built-in platform design. Whatever way it is accomplished, raising the client helps to save your back and for some reason clients equate the raised platform with a more professionally delivered service. Client safety must be your first consideration should you design your own custom elevated platform type of service area. Some raised pedicure setups have no handrail for the client to use when getting into or out of the pedicure chair. Some of these units are over 24 inches high! Sooner or later an accident will happen. It is much better to plan for safety than to be sorry later.

Considering the amount of dirty laundry generated by nail and foot services, the salon should have its own laundry area if possible. It saves hauling laundry to and from home if you do it yourself. It will also save money and be less expensive than a laundry service. The initial expense is small if one considers these two factors alone. Take, for example, the ultimate laundry at the Day Spa Beautique Salon in Houston, Texas. This is a large full service salon that generates large quantities of laundry. They have two separate laundry

Make sure that the foot baths and surrounding areas are sanitized and disinfected between each client.

rooms, each with a fully computerized washer and dryer. The operator needs only to place the laundry into the washer and punch in the code for the type of laundry being washed. The proper amount of soap and disinfectant is dispensed and the wash cycle is completed automatically. The laundry is then moved to the dryer where the process is completed. This is the ultimate setup! The Beautique Salon has 4000 square feet of space and serves many clients daily. The pedicure area alone has eight fully-plumbed pedicure spa chairs! To provide cost-effective quality service in this setting they need this type of laundry setup. For a small salon the small stackable washer and dryer sets will work well and will take up little room in a well-designed floor plan.

Other areas of a well planned salon will include a rest room, a supply room, and possibly an employee lounge. The size of these will depend on the individual salon. The main thing to remember is to keep these areas as clean and sanitary as the rest of the salon.

F O O T   N O T E S

Every time you enter your salon view it as a client would.

The salon is your home for a part of your life. Make it as pleasant for yourself as you can. Every time you enter your salon view it as a client would. It is a place where you make first impressions as well as lasting impressions on your clients. Remember this and see that they are impressed by the surroundings into which they have chosen to come. Design each room or work area so that it is elegant, uncluttered, and serviceable. Pedicure areas should be as private as possible. Seating for both you and your client must be comfortable and designed so that a service can be easily and comfortably provided. Above all, an easily accessible sink must be available for clients as well as yourself. Cleanliness and proper salon sanitation must be your number one priority. Take pride in your surroundings and reap the benefits.

QUESTIONS

1. Why are fungi, yeast, bacteria, and viruses more prevalent in the salon setting?

2. What are the definitions of sanitation, disinfection, and sterilization?

3. Define biocidal. Are disinfectants biocidal agents?

4. Name the five classes of disinfectants.

5. What is the most important factor affecting the action of disinfectants in your salon?

6. What is the beginning of the disinfection process?

7. How many times do you get to make a first impression on your clients?

8. Why is a pedestal type chair important for the pedicure?

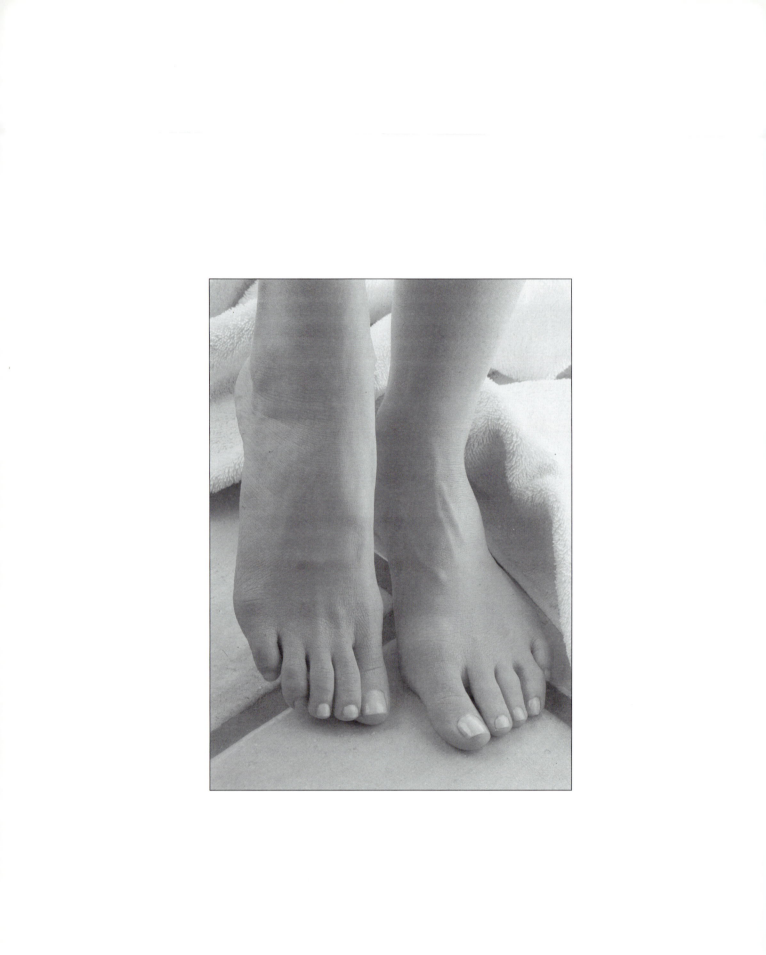

The Pedicure | 10

LEARNING OBJECTIVES

After studying this chapter, the reader should be able to:

1. Name a few groups of people who benefit greatly from having a pedicure.

2. Describe the three basic product classes used for the pedicure.

3. Describe products used to enhance the pedicure.

4. Relate the five basic steps of the pedicure and their functions.

5. Define the three basic forms of hand manipulation used in therapeutic message.

6. Describe the variations of massage technique used to massage the feet.

7. Define reflexology.

8. Describe the basic aim of reflexology and how to attain it.

9. Describe the training necessary to become a reflexologist.

OVERVIEW

The pedicure promotes foot health and is a part of good personal grooming. It should be the most relaxing, stress-reducing service a nail professional provides. The feeling of satisfaction and accomplishment the pedicurist receives after being able to make the client comfortable is exhilarating. A well performed pedicure promotes a sense of well-being and relaxation in the client. Once they experience it, clients will want to continue pedicure services on a routine basis. Satisfied pedicure clients will make follow-up pedicure appointments and refer others for your services. Promoted as "the healthy thing to do for your feet" and as a service that helps to prevent foot problems it will add income to the salon.

Society in general and many nail professionals may view the foot as an unclean part of our anatomy. This is far from the truth! Think about it. In our society daily bathing is the norm. We get up in the morning and take a bath or shower. We then put on clean undergarments, which in most cases includes hosiery. Our feet are then placed into shoes. This protects them further from the outside environment during our daily activities.

Our hands, however, are constantly in contact with everything around us. We are taught from early childhood to always cover our mouth if we cough. We use our hands to assist in bodily functions. We shake hands with others as a friendly greeting. We touch handrails, doorknobs, money, and many other objects that have been touched by many before us. Influenza, the common cold, and other diseases are transferred from one person to another through contact with the hands. Have you ever heard of anyone catching a cold from handling another person's foot?

Remind your clients that pedicures are for all seasons, not just special occasions!

Yes, feet do have their own peculiar odor caused from the byproducts of the normal flora that live on our feet. Its fragrance does not mean that the foot is unclean. Organisms that exist on our feet, under normal circumstances, will not live and multiply on our hands. For all of these reasons the nail professional should not consider the foot a dirty or unhealthy part of the client when providing a pedicure.

Pedicures should be promoted as the healthy thing to do for the feet. Likewise pedicures should also be promoted as a part of good grooming and as a preventive health aid. And pedicures also make you feel great! Pedicures are not just a summer thing to do for the feet. Nor are they just to make them look good when wearing open-toed shoes. However, some clients will come only for these reasons. It is your job as a nail professional to convince them otherwise. We do use our feet daily and they need routine maintenance to serve our needs.

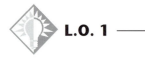 **L.O. 1**

The elderly also need care and maintenance for their feet on a year-round basis. This is called "routine foot care" by insurance companies and they will only pay for this under very strict guidelines. Those covered are people with diabetes, arteriosclerosis, and certain other severe medical problems that would make it dangerous for the nonmedically trained person (layperson) to work on the foot. Many elderly people cannot reach their feet and need help in caring for their feet. It is estimated that 40 million Americans suffer from some form of arthritis. Many of them cannot reach their feet and if they can, then they cannot squeeze the nail nippers. They need the foot care a good pedicurist can provide. The nail professional who offers pedicure services for these people, beside adding to their income, will be doing these individuals a great favor.

Among other individuals in our society who would particularly benefit from a pedicure service are joggers, dancers, and cosmetologists. These groups all are particularly dependent on their feet for their livelihood or enjoyment. Promotions directed at them will be well-received and are a great way of building a satisfied clientele. Do not forget the men! They make up about half of the population and once they experience the comfort and relaxation of a good pedicure they will return for more. Promotional activities directed at them are dollars well spent.

Not all clients will want or need a full pedicure service. Some only need a professional nail trimming. If you really analyze it, pedicure services are for everyone. Do not limit yourself. Tailor your pedicure service to meet the needs of the entire population. Be creative and enjoy the financial rewards and satisfactions that come by providing a professional pedicure.

The previous chapters have covered those conditions of the foot under which a foot service should or should not be provided by the nail professional. The following discussion assumes that a history and personal evaluation have been performed, and that the nail professional has recognized any abnormal conditions that may be present and has made the decision to proceed with the pedicure service. Now is the time to have some fun!

If you really analyze it, pedicure services are for everyone. Do not limit yourself.

FOOT NOTES

Pedicures are a part of good grooming but most of all they promote foot health. The client looks forward to and expects the pedicure to be a relaxing and stress-reducing experience. Beauty is an added secondary benefit. The pedicurist must meet these expectations by mastering the techniques of the professional pedicure.

Feet are not dirty! They all have their own individual personalities and appearances. Become acquainted with your clients' feet and experience with them the satisfaction of a pedicure.

All segments of our society will benefit from a pedicure. Be creative and promote pedicures to fit the individual needs of each. Proper promotion will add to your income and increase your client base. Most of all have fun!

L.O. 2

We have discussed what instruments and equipment are necessary to perform the pedicure. Now let us discuss the products you will need to perform the professional pedicure. At least three basic product classes are necessary for the pedicure service. These consist of soaks, scrubs, and massage products.

Soaks

These are products used in the pedicure bath to soften the skin of the foot. A good soak should contain an **antiseptic** to sanitize the foot, moisturizers or **hydrating** agents, and a **surfactant** to reduce the surface tension of the tissues and allow for deeper penetration of the active ingredients. Dead Sea salts are one of the ingredients often found in the better soaking agents. Because large amounts of therapeutic minerals such as potassium, magnesium, calcium, and sodium are found in them, they contribute to superhydration of the skin. They also contain **antioxidants**, which help to counterbalance the surfactants that can be harsh to the skin.

Natural antiseptics such as **tea tree oil** may be used as well as other antiseptic agents. If a soap is used it should be gentle on the skin. It should have more of a shampoo quality rather than that of a harsh cleaner. Other natural oils may be used for their moisturizing and **aromatherapy** qualities. The soak really sets the stage for the rest of the pedicure. Be sure to purchase one that meets all the requirements necessary to start the pedicure off on the right foot, so to speak.

Use the correct products to start your pedicure services on the right foot!

Scrubs

These are used to help in the removal and smoothing of the dry flaky skin and callus that build up on the foot. The scrub should be abrasive to do the job. However, it should not be too abrasive so that it will remove the living skin from the hands of the pedicurist who will be using it repeatedly. A good scrub will contain more softening agents such as **alpha-hydroxy acids** (AHA), or oils to further soften and penetrate the nonliving areas of skin that need removal. The scrub will also contain an **exfoliating** agent which acts as an abrasive. This helps to mechanically remove the desired nonliving tissue. Sea sand, ground apricot kernels, pumice, quartz crystals, and plastic beads are all exfoliating agents found in pedicure scrubs. Agents such as **glycerin** are also found in scrubs. These tend to bind with the flakes of tissue and assist in pulling them off the underlying living skin during the exfoliating process. Paraffin, cornmeal, or oatmeal may also serve the same purpose. Vitamins, essential aroma oils, and other moisturizers that help to condition the skin may also be found in the various scrub preparations.

Massage Preparations

Massage oils are used to lubricate, moisturize, and invigorate the skin. They allow the hands of the pedicurist to glide soothingly over the skin during the massage part of the pedicure. They also help to promote a general feeling of relaxation and well-being in the client. A quality massage oil will not absorb into the skin too fast. The **molecular** size of the oil determines the rate of absorption. Lanolin and mineral oil are examples of large **molecule** oils. Most quality massage oils are a blend of therapeutic oils that promote skin health. Jojoba oil and vitamin E oil are examples. Aromatherapy oils may also be incorporated for their relaxing and calming effects. Tea tree oil is often included for its antiseptic and antifungal qualities. Glycerine or **silicone** may also be added to help lower the friction coefficient. Pedicurists, as do some massage therapists, may want to formulate their own massage oil. Some massage therapy supply stores have base massage oils to which different essential or aromatherapy oils can be added. A number of different massage oils may be formulated in this manner to match individual client needs. This will give a customized quality to the pedicure.

Massage lotions have smaller molecules and thus are fast absorbing. They may be used at the end of the massage to further moisturize and invigorate the skin. They may contain AHA preparations and essential oils, all of which promote skin health and longevity. Properly formulated they may help to retard the growth of callus. Tea tree, vitamin E, jojoba, and other similar oils are also often part of the formulation found in massage lotions.

Add-on Products

These are products offered to enhance and expedite the pedicure experience. Various high-intensity callus softeners are offered to help soften and remove the excess callus that builds up around the heels and over pressure points. A 20% AHA preparation is an example of this. It is applied directly to the callus and allowed to soak in and soften the excess callus buildup. This makes the callus easier to remove with the exfoliates and callus paddles.

——— **L.O. 3**

Masks composed of mineral clays, sea extracts, hydrating AHA, aromatherapy oils, and other therapeutic skin softeners give the feet a special "mud facial" experience. These seem to be excellent products and clients really enjoy them.

Hot paraffin baths for the feet are also an excellent addition to the pedicure. They open the pores of the skin allowing for penetration of essential oils that are incorporated within the paraffin. The paraffin bath also stimulates circulation and the deep heat produced helps to reduce inflammation and promote circulation to the affected joints. Aromatherapy oils are also incorporated into the bath. Clients feel pampered and the hot wax service adds to the relaxation of the pedicure experience. **WARNING:** Do not give this service to clients with impaired circulation, loss of feeling, or other diabetic-related problems. The hot wax may cause burns or skin breakdown in these situations.

Pedicure Systems or Lines. These are available from many manufacturers of professional nail products. Five quality systems are manufactured by Beautiful Feet®, Creative Nail Design Systems®, Gena® Laboratories®, and Salon Systems®. These manufacturers all produce a complete line of products for the professional pedicure. If you are just starting to offer pedicures check out these lines and any others that interest you. Compare them with each other and decide for yourself what is the best for your clients. Put the educational support and commitment of the company on the top of the list in making a decision. Those companies that offer classes and training in the use of their line will be available when you have specific questions about individual client problems or their lines in general. There are also new products being offered all the time so be sure to keep up on the latest information available.

Know the product lines available for providing pedicure services to your clients.

PEDICURE PROCEDURE

Manufacturers of each pedicure line offer a step-by-step customized procedure to be followed when using their products. If using their products, follow their procedures. They have been tested and found to enhance the effectiveness of their product line. For economic reasons you should time the individual steps of the pedicure so that it takes approximately an hour to complete the entire service. Do not give the client the feeling of being rushed but develop your procedures so you have no wasted motions. To do this you must be as comfortable as the client. You have already begun this by selecting the equipment that fits your height and work requirements. Have your instruments and products within easy reach. Have warm dry towels available to dry and place the foot on when it is not in the bath.

There should be no distractions for you or the client during the pedicure.

Be "one" with your client. There should be no distractions for you or the client during the pedicure. You should at all times during the pedicure know what your client needs and desires from you as far as the service is concerned. Make your clients feel that you have nothing more to do but to take care of their every wish. Talk to them if they want to talk but if they want to drift off into another place give them the peace and tranquility they are looking for.

Be gentle but firm when handling the foot. A gentle light touch or hold will produce a tickling sensation, which is not relaxing. The client will become tense and pull away from the pedicurist during the service. How many people have you heard say that they cannot stand having their feet touched? A firm but comfortable grip on the foot will help to overcome this problem. In most instances when working on the foot is should be grasped at the midtarsal area between the thumb and fingers. This accomplishes two things. It locks the foot making it rigid instead of being flexible and loose. It also allows the placing of the thumb or index finger, depending on which foot you are working on, at that point on the plantar aspect where the two skin creases on the ball meet. This spot is usually located at the beginning of the longitudinal arch. Applying varying degrees of pressure to this point seems to have a calming effect on clients and overcomes any apprehension they may have about someone touching their feet (Figure 10-1).

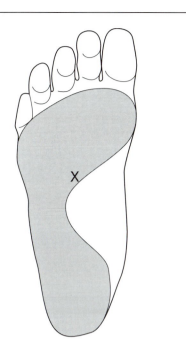

Figure 10-1 X marks the spot. Applying pressure to this area on a ticklish or apprehensive client will have a calming effect.

The actual performance of the pedicure can be divided into five basic steps—the soak, nail care, skin care, massage, and polishing the nails. Each of these steps is distinct from the other. Depending on client needs some steps may not be necessary. For example, some clients may only need nail care. This should take no more than 15 minutes and all of the other steps of the full pedicure may be dispensed with. Yes, you can omit the soak. If it is included the nail service will take more time and therefore you should charge for it. If you have a great massage technique clients may want only the soak and a massage to relieve tension and stress after a day's work. Remember, be innovative and creative when it comes to your pedicure services. Now let's discuss a full service professional pedicure.

——— **L.O. 4**

The Soak

This procedure starts the service. It is important for softening and preparing the skin for what is to follow. It sets the stage for what is to come. The water should be around 104°F. If the client's circulation is compromised it should not be over 100°F. Place the soaking product into the water according to manufacturer's recommendation. Allow the client to soak for approximately 10 minutes. This sanitizes the foot and begins the removal of dry skin and callus. You have time during this part of the service to make sure everything you will need for the rest of the pedicure is where it should be. You do not want to stop and hunt for something during the pedicure process.

Innovation and creativity will enhance your pedicure services.

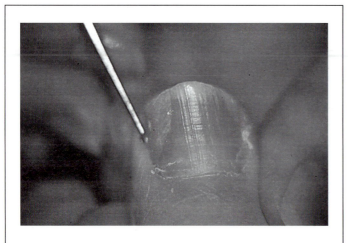

Figure 10-2 *The curette being used as an extension of the fingers to gently push the soft tissue away from the nail margin.*

Nail Care

This should follow soaking. Remove one foot from the bath and dry it with a towel. At this point an application of the callus softeners to any areas of excess dry skin or callus buildup on the foot as well as to the cuticle areas is recommended. This will give the product time to work while you care for the nails. After application of the callus softener use the curette, as an extension of the fingers, to gently push the soft tissue folds away from the lateral nail walls (Figure 10-2). This allows you to visually inspect the nail so that it can be trimmed without injuring the client. If there is extra buildup along the margin that blocks your view of the nail, it should be gently removed with the curette.

Using the toenail nippers as described in Chapter 8, the nails should now be carefully trimmed. The nippers are used like a pair of scissors (Figure 10-3). The nail is trimmed in a number of small cuts so as not to flatten it out and injure the hyponychium. Place the nipper over the free nail edge and slightly tilt the top of the nipper back toward the nail plate. This reduces the possibility of cutting the soft tissue hyponychium. Give the nipper a slight squeeze before actually cutting the nail. The reaction of the client to this squeeze will tell you if you are cutting too deep. If you get a reaction, reposition the nipper on the nail and start the process again.

In most instances you will trim the lesser toenails straight across and then remove the small sharp corners. This can be done later with the file if they do not turn down into the soft tissue margins. The big toenail is usually the most challenging to trim. The nail margins, in most instances, turn down into the nail groove and as a result soft tissue debris, lint, soap, and other material buildup occurs. Trim the great toenail just as described for the lesser toes but then pay particular attention to the nail margins. Gently slip the point of the nipper under the sharp corner of the margin and trim it off at about a 45° angle (Figure 10-4). Remember not to trim it back too far. If you do, you will leave a hook on the nail margin. If you can see the fine point of the nipper extending slightly beyond the edge of the nail before you cut it,

Always use great care when trimming toenails.

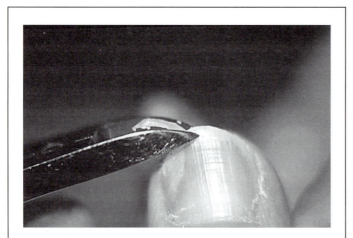

Figure 10-3 *The nail nippers are used like a pair of scissors making a number of small cuts across the nail.*

you should not get into trouble. If you do leave a hook, it must be removed. Otherwise an infection will most likely occur when the sharp point penetrates the soft tissue. If the hook is not deep in the margin, gently remove it with the nipper. If it is difficult to remove with the nipper move on to the next step and remove it with the small nail file or curette.

After the nails have been trimmed with the nipper go back to the curette and gently remove any debris left along the nail margins. This is done by placing the cupped part of the curette against the lateral nail wall and edge of the nail. Gently draw the curette along the nail. This process may have to be repeated a number of times. In most instances this will remove an adequate amount of the nonliving debris from the nail margins thus relieving the pressure and making the client comfortable. During this process also check the nail margins for rough areas and any hooks that may have been left behind after the trimming.

The curette is also used to remove dry cuticle from the top of the nail plate. The cuticle at the eponychium should not be pushed back on toenails. Any small break in the seal created by the true cuticle attachment to the nail plate at this level will allow fungal or bacterial infections to occur. To remove the cuticle from the top of the nail, the curette is drawn over the plate away from the eponychium in a sweeping "C" motion (Figure 10-5). You will need to repeat this motion a number of times to remove all of the cuticle debris from the top of the nail plate. WARNING: Be careful not to injure the eponychium during this process.

The small nail rasp is then used to smooth off the edges of the nail margins along the nail grooves (Figure 10-6). The rasp is made for this purpose. It is narrow and will only file the nail in one direction. It can be used to remove, smooth, and round off any sharp

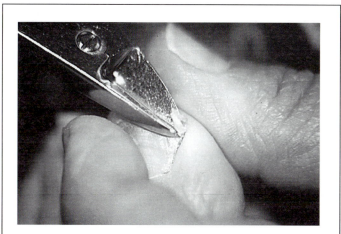

Figure 10-4 *Trim the nail at a 45° angle. Notice the tilt of the nipper to reduce the possibility of injury to the underlying soft tissue.*

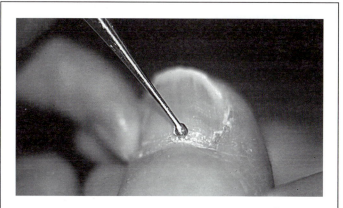

Figure 10-5 *The curette is also used to remove the dead cuticle on the top of the nail plate. A C motion is used as described in the text.*

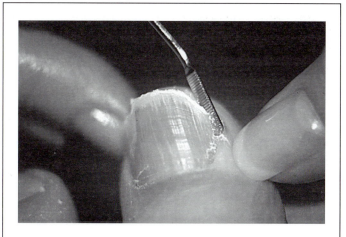

Figure 10-6 *The small nail file or rasp is used to gently smooth off the nail margin removing any rough edges or hooks left behind after the trimming process.*

points that may be present along these margins. Do not use it as a probe but gently draw it along the edge of that portion of the nail that you have just trimmed. Small short strokes with the file will accomplish the task.

The diamond file should then be used to finally shape and smooth the rest of the nail. If the nail is thick, the file is also used to thin the nail plate. This file is used in the same manner as you use your regular nail files. Because of its construction the diamond file can be easily sanitized and kept in the disinfectant solution. If you do not have a diamond file you may use the regular nail files that you use for fingernail services. The problem is that these files cannot really be disinfected. Literature states most disinfectants must be in contact with the fungal organisms we find in toenails for a number of hours to destroy them. The regular nail files are not made to be in the disinfectants for this long a dwell time.

If some of the nails are thick you may use an electric drill to mechanically reduce the thickness. WARNING: *You should only use the drill if you have had hands-on training in its use. This training must be provided by someone who is qualified and knowledgeable about the use of the drill for thinning the toenail.* A salesperson is usually not qualified to give this training. The drill used by a qualified nail professional is a safe time-saving tool when it comes to thinning a thick toenail.

After completing the nail service on one foot replace it in the soak and repeat the process described above on the other foot. The entire nail trimming process should take approximately 15 minutes.

Skin Care

Care of the skin is the next step in the full service pedicure. The skin has been softened by the soaking solution. The thicker areas of dry skin and callus have been softened with the extra strength callus softeners during the nail trimming procedure. The exfoliative scrubbing product is now used to reduce and remove the unwanted skin. One foot is removed from the bath and the scrub is liberally applied to the foot. Using a massaging type of motion the pedicurist scrubs the dry skin off the foot. Pay particular attention using extra friction on the heels and other areas where more callus and dry skin builds up. During this process the abrasive foot paddle is used to smooth and thin more of the thicker areas of callus. Remember callus protects the underlying skin from irritation and is there for a purpose. Remove only enough to make the client comfortable. WARNING: *Calluses should be smoothed not removed.* You may need to educate your client about callus formation and the protective function it provides. The foot is then rinsed off in the bath. Do not forget to clean between the toes. These areas are often missed.

Callus on your client's foot has a purpose — to protect the underlying skin. Smooth, but do not remove, the callus!

If a mask product is to be used this is the time to use it. After rinsing and cleaning the foot, apply the mask according to manufacturer's recommendations. Wrap the foot in a clean towel and rest it on the footrest. The scrubbing process is then completed on the other foot. The scrubbing process should take approximately 10 minutes. At this point approximately 35 minutes have been used for the pedicure. You may wish to allow the client to relax with the mask product for another 5 minutes. This will leave 20 minutes for the massage and polish.

The hot wax service may be added at this point in the pedicure. It may be used in place of the mask or as a separate add-on part of the pedicure. The wax should be applied in accordance with manufacturer's instructions. A plastic baggy is then placed over the wax and then the foot is wrapped in a towel. The process is repeated on the other foot and the client should then be allowed to relax in silence for 5 to 10 minutes. This allows for the penetration of the heat and oils from the wax into the skin and underlying tissues. It can also be a nice prelude to the massage. Remember this is an add-on service that takes more time and requires special equipment; therefore, it warrants an extra charge.

The Massage

The **massage** is that part of the professional pedicure where the nail professional can excel. This is what the client has been looking forward to. A good massage will make the client come back for the next pedicure. The nail professional who perfects a good massage technique will not lack pedicure clients. Relaxation is the most important part of the massage. It will give the client a feeling of well-being and exhilaration. The massage also promotes increased circulation and muscle relaxation within the lower extremities.

Massage is defined in the medical dictionary as "a method of manipulation of the body by rubbing, pinching, kneading, tapping, etc." Touch is the first of our senses to develop and under normal circumstances the last to diminish. Babies in the first few months of life receive most stimuli and information about their surroundings through the sense of touch. The frail 90-year-old who may be losing his sight will still receive sensations of joy and well-being through the loving touch of a friend or relative. Most of us enjoy being touched and the art of massage takes touching to a higher level.

There are three basic forms of hand **manipulation** used in therapeutic massage. These consist of:

◆ Light or hard stroking movements called **effleurage**

◆ Compression movements called **pétrissage**, which includes kneading, squeezing and friction

A good massage will make the client come back for the next pedicure.

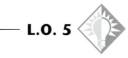 L.O. 5

◆ Percussion or **tapotement**, where the sides of the hands are used to strike the skin and underlying tissues in rapid succession

Effleurage relaxes muscles and improves circulation to the small surface blood vessels. It also increases blood flow toward the heart. Pétrissage helps to increase movement by stretching muscles, tendons, and any scar tissue present from previous injuries. Tapotement is also a technique for improving circulation. For the pedicure massage effleurage and pétrissage are the two basic manipulations used. Listed below are some variations of all three techniques:

L.O. 6 ⸻

1. **Relaxer movement to the joint of the foot:** Rest client's foot on footrest or stool. Grasp the leg just above the ankle with your left hand. This will brace the client's leg and foot. Use your right hand to hold left foot just beneath toes and rotate foot in a circular motion.

2. **Effleurage on top of foot:** Place both thumbs on top of foot at instep. Move your thumbs in circular movements in opposite directions down the center of the top of the foot. Continue this movement to the toes. Keep one hand in contact with foot or leg, slide one hand at a time back firmly to instep and rotate back down toes. This is a relaxing movement. Repeat three to five times.

3. **Effleurage on heel:** Use the same thumb movement that you did in the massage technique above. Start at the base of the toes and move from the ball of the foot to the heel, rotating your thumbs in opposite directions. Slide hands back to the top of foot. This is a relaxing movement. Repeat three to five times.

4. **Effleurage movement on toes:** Start with the little toe, using thumb on top and index finger on bottom of foot. Hold each toe and rotate with thumb. Start at base of toe and work toward the end of the toes. This is relaxing and soothing. Repeat three to five times.

5. **Joint movement for toes:** Start with little toe and make a figure eight with each toe. Repeat three to five times.

6. **Thumb compression—friction movement:** Make a fist with your fingers, keeping your thumb out. Apply firm pressure with your thumb and move your fist up the heel toward the ball of the foot. Work from the left side of foot and back down the right side toward the heel. As you massage over the bottom of the foot, check for any nodules or bumps. If you find one, be very gentle because the area may be tender. This movement stimulates the blood flow and increases circulation.

For the pedicure massage effleurage and pétrissage are the two basic manipulations used.

7. Metatarsal scissors (a pétrissage movement, kneading): Place your fingers on top of foot along metatarsal bones with your thumb underneath the foot. Knead up and down along each bone by raising your thumb and lower fingers to apply pressure. This promotes flexibility and stimulates blood flow. Repeat three to five times.

8. Fist twist compression (a friction movement, deep rubbing): Place your left hand on top of foot and make a fist with your right hand. Your left hand will apply pressure while your right hand twists around the bottom of the foot. This helps stimulate blood flow. Repeat three to five times up and around foot.

9. Effleurage on instep: Place fingers at ball of foot. Move fingers in circular movements in opposite directions. Massage to end of each toe, gently squeezing the tip of each toe.

10. Percussion or tapotement movement: Use fingertips to perform percussion or tapotement movements to lightly tap over the entire foot to reduce blood circulation and complete massage.

There are any number of massage styles and techniques. Numerous books have been written on the various forms and styles of massage. Study them and develop your own expertise. No two individuals will have the same massage technique. However, no matter what technique you use perfect it so that it becomes second nature to you. A basic massage therapy course from a massage school will be money well spent. Study and practice different methods so that you can individualize the massage for different clients. During this part of the pedicure, be keenly aware of your clients' needs and meet those requirements by giving a massage that fulfills them.

Attention to the fine details will make your massage stand out from others.

Della Perry, of the Mueller College of Holistic Studies in San Diego, says it best when she states, "Keep a smile in your hands—think about your touch and imagine how good you would like it to feel." She also recommends that the pressure of the massage be applied only as deeply as is comfortable for you and your client. Ask the client whether she would like more or less pressure. Be aware of what areas or parts of the massage the client enjoys most and work those areas more. Work toward the heart to facilitate circulation. Keep your wrists straight to reduce stress and strain on yourself. Do not favor your dominant hand, always remembering to alternate the pressures from one to the other. Attention to the fine details will make your massage stand out from others.

Apply Nail Polish (Optional)

After the massage, if the client desires, nail polish may be applied according to the manufacturer's recommendations. While you are doing this you may want to recommend take-home products for the client to use between pedicures. Ask the client what she liked or disliked about the pedicure and note it on the client record after she has gone. Also talk about the next appointment and set up the client's next pedicure. Once the client has left, sanitize the equipment and instruments that were used and then place the instruments back into the disinfectant solution. You are now ready for your next pedicure client.

FOOT NOTES

Three basic classes of products are necessary to provide the professional pedicure: soaks, scrubs, and massage oils or lotions. Different manufacturers provide them either individually or as a pedicure product line. Choose the products carefully. Purchase them from a manufacturer who has demonstrated excellence in providing education and service for the product.

The pedicure consists of five basic parts plus add-on services. These basic parts are soaking, toenail care, scrubbing or exfoliation, massage, and nail polish (optional). Added services may include mud masks, and hot wax treatments. Perfect each part of the service, particularly the massage. A good massage will make the client want to come back for more. Always remember, it is your attention to detail that will make the foot service you provide stand out from the rest.

REFLEXOLOGY

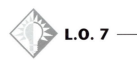 **L.O. 7**

Reflexology is the precise manipulation of the nerve endings in the hands and feet to stimulate the body's organs, nerves, and glands. The beauty industry, particularly the nails section of the industry, has become very interested in the practice of reflexology. We are seeing more nail professionals offering a "reflexology service or massage" as a part of their services. Reflexology has made itself a place in the healing arts. Used as an adjunct with other conventional medical treatments it relieves stress, reduces pain, and promotes healing. The true practice of reflexology is not to be taken lightly.

No one culture can claim to have originated reflexology. History shows that different cultures from all over the world, since the beginning of time, have found that **reflexes** affect the health of individuals. The relationship of the feet (and hands) to the internal organs of the body has been recognized by many different cultures since before recorded history. Pictures of the practice of foot massage are all we find that may depict the earliest recordings of this practice.

Egyptian **pictographs** depict foot care whether it be massage, reflexology, or the care of a malady of the great toe. This is 2500 BC! The Egyptians were the first to study medicine. Reflexology probably migrated from Egypt to Greece and Arabia. Then it moved to Europe after Egypt was conquered by Alexander the Great. Manuscripts preserved from that time tend to support this theory.

Five thousand years ago in India reflexology was also known. Buddhist monks brought it to China and from there it moved to Japan. Indian drawings depict areas of the feet that relate to various parts of the body. Some of these drawings also depict foot massage (or was it reflexology?). In 618 to 907 AD a Japanese monk brought to Japan the **Soku Shinjutsu** (observation of the feet and treatment of the foot nerves) art of reflexology. China called this "Examining the Foot Method." This was 4000 years ago and it was used as a part of **acupuncture**. Marco Polo and missionaries brought to Europe from China the Chinese version of foot reflexology thus joining the Egyptian and Chinese techniques. **Zone therapy** was the result. Zone therapy states that pressures applied to particular zones of the body will cause a beneficial reflex action in another part of the same zone.

During the Dark Ages research and advancement in medicine and science stalled. Not until the 1880s did the specialty of **neurology** come into being. Many scientific papers published by the British on the relationship of a reflex action and the cure of disease were recorded and in the 1890s and early 1900s, German physicians developed reflex massage. They associated positive reactions in other parts of the body when pressure was applied to areas of the body that were painful. In 1929, the physical therapist Elisabeth Dicke developed connective tissue massage based on reflex zone massage.

The Incas and American Indians also used various forms of foot reflexology. Little is known about its origin or practice in these areas. About 1909, 10 zones of the body were "rediscovered" by Dr. Fitzgerald of the United States. He stated that working anywhere in the zone affected all areas of the zone. He tried to teach his zone therapy to medical doctors but was rebuffed by the organized medical establishment. Because of the controversial nature of this subject among his medical colleagues, Fitzgerald was forced to take his knowledge to **chiropractors**, **naturopaths**, **osteopaths**, dentists, and the general public.

Believing in Fitzgerald's work, Dr. Joe Selby Reiley was the first in America to draw detailed diagrams of the reflex zones of the foot, hands, and ears. He also added to Fitzgerald's work by describing eight horizontal zones in the body. In the early 1930s, Eunice Ingham, a lay person, worked under Dr. Reiley as his therapist. She was instrumental in separating zone therapy from reflexes of the feet. She worked with doctors to prove to them that reflexology was a useful diagnostic tool. She made two major contributions to

History shows that different cultures from all over the world have found that reflexes affect the health of individuals.

reflexology as we know it today. First, she found that alternating pressure had a stimulating effect rather than a numbing effect. Second, she took the knowledge to the public by giving extensive lectures throughout the United States. She also published books on reflexology, which were extensively circulated among the lay population. She is the one who gave reflexology credibility in the United States.

In the 1950s, reflexology came under attack by organized medicine who tried to label it as practicing medicine without a license. Reflexology in some states may be practiced for relaxation purposes only. Currently there is a resurgence of public interest in alternative and complementary health practices. Reflexology again has come to the forefront of public awareness. True reflexologists of today believe that they practice a complementary therapy rather than an alternative therapy. Alternative implies that the practice is better than, or an alternative to, or replaces other forms of treatment when in fact it does not.

Some believe that as a complement to traditional medical care reflexology aids in stress reduction and pain control

There is also more acceptance of reflexology methods today in some circles of modern medicine. Some believe that as a complement to traditional medical care reflexology aids in stress reduction and pain control. In Hospice programs for terminally ill cancer patients reflexology has aided in pain control and stress reduction and enhanced the quality of life during their final days. In addition, many podiatrists offer a certified reflexologist who is available to provide services for patients.

It seems to be impossible to give a rational explanation of why reflexology works. Part of it is an art learned over many years of practice. The other part is a full knowledge and understanding of anatomy and physiology of the human body and how these areas may be affected by reflexology techniques. The terms reflexology and foot massage should not be interchanged. Foot massage implies rubbing and kneading of the tissues of the foot in general. Reflexology is the more precise application of pressure to specific reflex points located on the foot. This application of pressure affects, through reflex action, the internal organs and other areas of the body some distance from the foot.

Briefly, the following are examples of different kinds of reflexes. One is blushing if you have been embarrassed. In this reflex the small blood vessels in the skin dilate (open up) as the result of an external stimulus affecting areas of the brain. This transmits a signal to the blood vessels in the skin telling them to dilate, which then allows more blood to rush into the area. Another simple reflex is pulling the finger away from a hot surface. This is done without any active thought process whatsoever. It is called a protective reflex.

Too much stimulation, whether internal or external, which results in overreaction, may do more harm than good. Take the case of "battle fatigue." Overstimulation of the individual to the stress of battle will cause a reflex within the body. A brain reflex begins to shut reactive processes down completely. This shutdown reflex gives the body a rest from the outside stimulus. This then allows a healing process to occur. Reflexes are powerful and should not to be dealt with lightly!

One of the primary aims of the reflexologist is to promote relaxation so that the body can heal itself. The reflexologist therefore must never "break contact" with the client. This means not only physically but also mentally. The reflexologist must at all times, when with the client, be cognizant of the wants, desires, and needs of that client. Author and reflexologist Christine Issel states, "Reflexology is a creative art and requires the hard work, practice and devotion that all forms of creativity do. Therefore, it is important when approaching reflexology, that the practitioner have an understanding of man's true nature and a belief in the healing techniques chosen for use."[1] Those nail professionals who are committed to this precept and are willing to devote the time and study necessary may call themselves reflexologists.

Reflexologists in many states have organized reflexology associations. There is a consensus among them that a national certification organization is a necessity. This organization would help to set standards for education in the field and ensure the competency of practitioners. To meet this need the American Reflexology Certification Board™[2] was created in 1991. This board does not replace certification programs offered by individual schools of reflexology. Its primary aim is to certify competency of reflexologists, who wish to practice as such, on a national basis. To meet the testing prerequisites the candidate must complete a hands-on reflexology course involving a minimum of 110 hours of hands-on instruction. Fifty-five of these hours must be instruction on anatomy and physiology, general and localized to the extremities, because these subjects correlate to the practice of reflexology. Also one must document 90 sessions (three per client) of actual hands-on reflexology. This makes for a total of 200 hours. Some states have already enacted legislation and developed regulations concerning reflexology. In April 1993, North Dakota became the first state to license reflexologists and establish a reflexology board. Other states are also considering the regulation of the practice of reflexology.

So what does this all mean as far as the overall care of the foot is concerned? The practice of reflexology through the ages has been refined and advanced to the point of being an acceptable complementary adjunct to the healing arts. For people to hold themselves up as practitioners of reflexology, they must be able to demonstrate a competent knowledge of anatomy and

—————— **L.O. 8**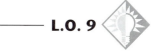

—————— **L.O. 9**

One of the primary aims of the reflexologist is to promote relaxation so that the body can heal itself.

---

[1] Issel, Christine, *Reflexology: Art, Science, & History*, New Frontier Publishing, P.O. Box 245855, Sacramento, CA 95824.

[2] American Reflexology Certification Board, P.O. Box 620607, Littleton, CO 80162, phone 303-6921, FAX 303-904-0460.

Mastery of massage techniques separates the good pedicurist from the master pedicurist.

physiology. They must also be able to demonstrate a satisfactory educational background in the subject of reflexology that would then allow them to safely give a reflexology service to clients. Hours of instruction in the theory and practice of reflexology are needed before competency as a reflexologist is attained. A weekend of instruction for certification is insufficient. Reflexology is not just an added service to increase revenues within a nail salon or podiatrist's office.

The massage part of the pedicure is what most clients will look forward to. Mastery of massage techniques separates the good pedicurist from the master pedicurist. Reflexology may be incorporated into the massage if the pedicurist has some expertise in those techniques. However, unless the pedicurist meets the knowledge requirements in anatomy and physiology and has the adequate training and background in hands-on reflexology technique she should not call herself a reflexologist by charging extra for a reflexology service. Until all of these requirements are met the pedicurist is only giving a "reflexology-like" massage. This is an integral part of the pedicure, not an add-on service.

FOOT NOTES

Reflexology is a precise system of manipulating the nerve endings of the feet and hands, thereby causing a change in the organs, nerves, and glands of the body. Reflexology is a science as well as an acquired art. It induces relaxation, increases circulation, and reduces pain thereby improving the healing potential of the body. A full understanding of anatomy and physiology is necessary for the provision of a professional reflexology service. An individual who is willing to devote the time to acquire the necessary educational background and training may call themself a reflexologist.

QUESTIONS

1. Who can benefit from a pedicure service?

2. What are the three basic product classes needed for a professional pedicure service?

3. Name two reasons why people should receive pedicures.

4. What should be the temperature of the water bath for soaking the feet?

5. How much callus should be removed during the pedicure?

6. The massage promotes a general feeling of well-being and relaxation. Name two other benefits of the massage within the lower extremity.

7. What is the difference between effleurage and pétrissage? What is the purpose of each of these hand manipulations in the massage?

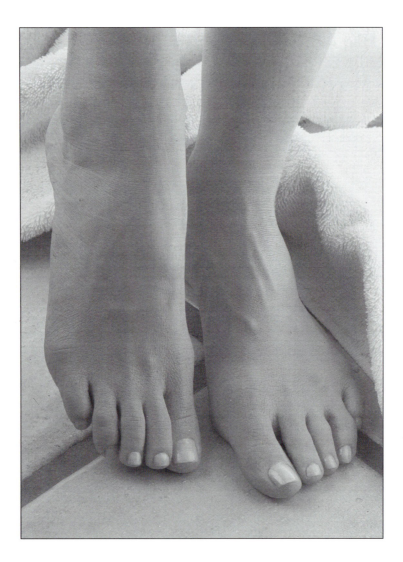

the salon professional's guide to
FOOT CARE

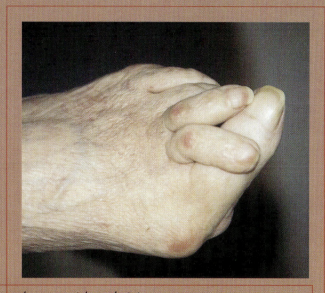

Rheumatoid Arthritis [Fig. 3-1]

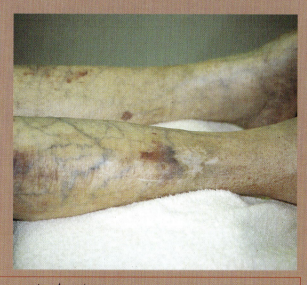

Arteriosclerosis [Fig. 3-5]

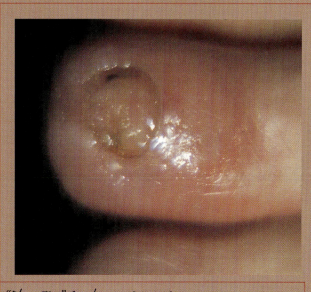

"Blue Toe" Syndrome [Fig. 3-6]

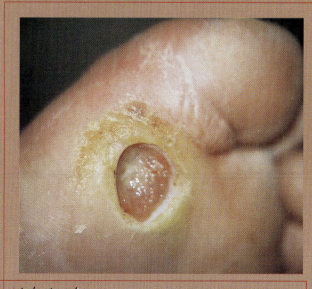

Diabetic Ulcer [Fig. 3-7]

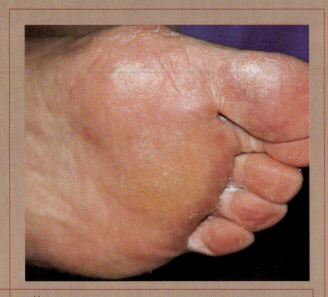

Callus [Fig. 4-5]

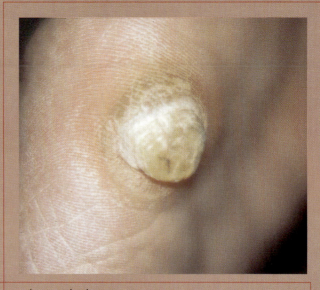

Indurated Plantar Keratoma [Fig. 4-6]

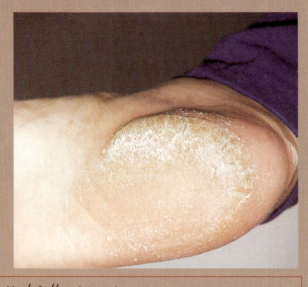

Heel Callus [Fig. 4-7]

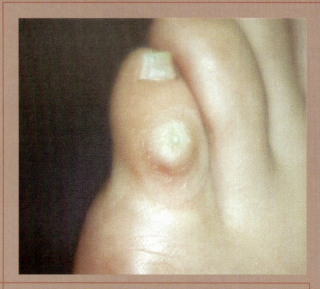

Hard Corn (Heloma Durum) [Fig. 4-8]

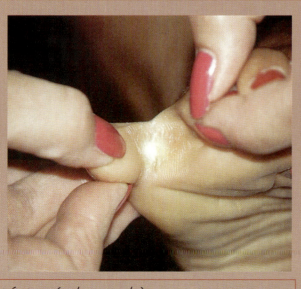

Soft Corn (Heloma Mole) [Fig. 4-9]

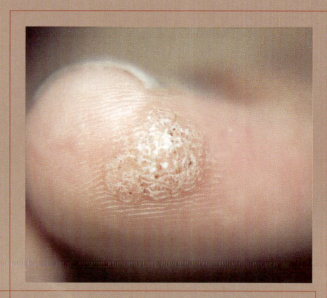

Warts [Fig. 4-10]

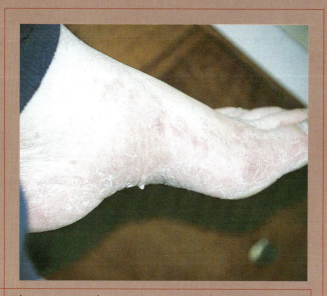

Chronic Hyperkeratotic Tinea Pedis [Fig. 4-11]

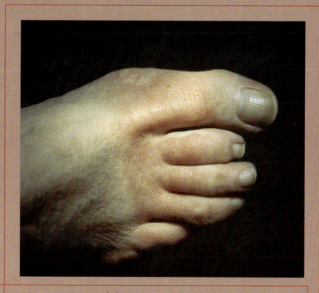

Contact Dermatitis [Fig. 4-12]

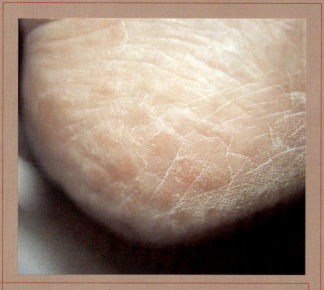

Piezogenic Papules [Fig. 4-13]

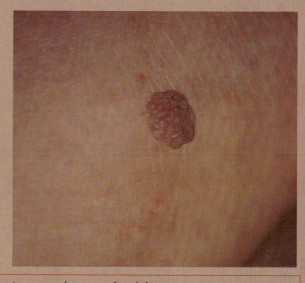

Pigmented Nevus (Mole) [Fig. 4-14]

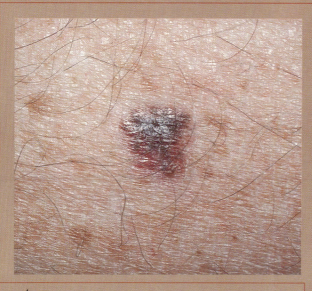

Melanoma [Fig. 4-15]

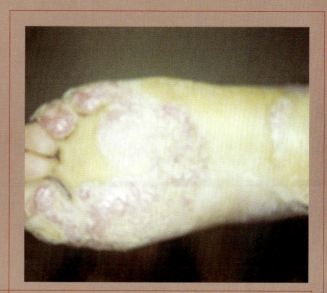

Psoriasis [Fig. 4-16]

3

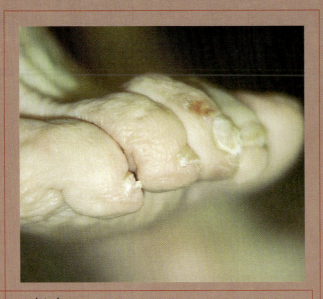

Multiple Hammertoe [Fig. 4-17]

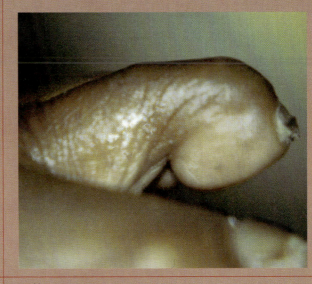

Mallet Toe [Fig. 4-18]

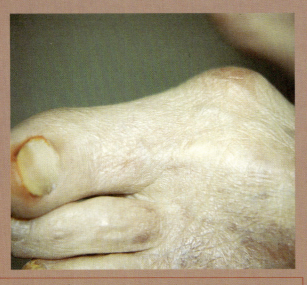

Hallux Valgus [Fig. 4-20]

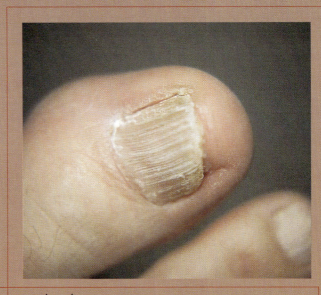

Onychorrhexis [Fig. 5-6]

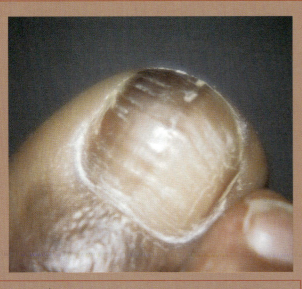

Beau's Lines [Fig. 5-7]

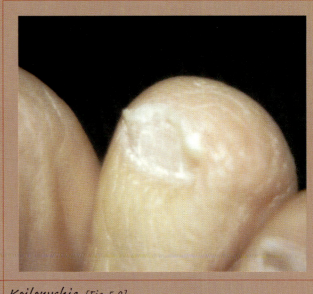

Koilonychia [Fig. 5-8]

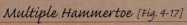

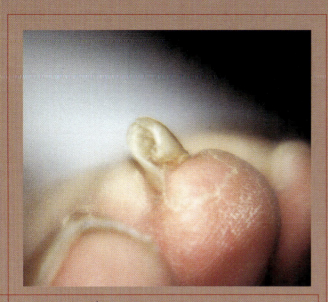

Trumpet Nail *[Fig. 5-9]*

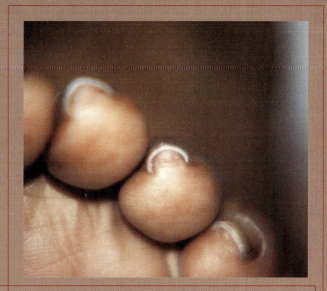

Tile-shaped Nails *[Fig. 5-10]*

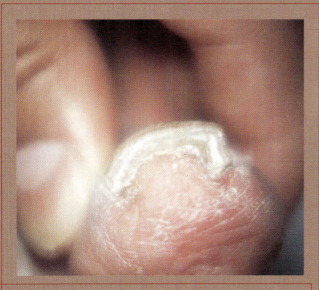

Plicatured Nail *[Fig. 5-11]*

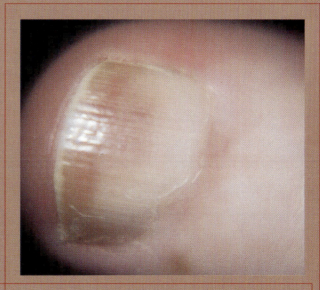

Pterygium *[Fig. 5-12]*

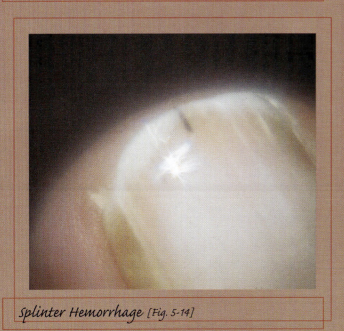

Splinter Hemorrhage *[Fig. 5-14]*

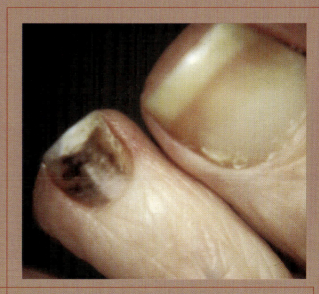

Subungual Hematoma (Blood Clot) *[Fig. 5-15]*

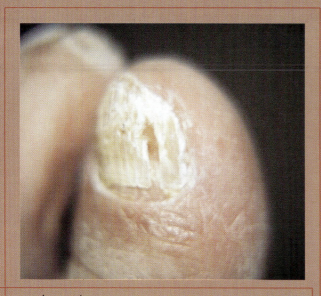

Onychomadesis [Fig. 5-16]

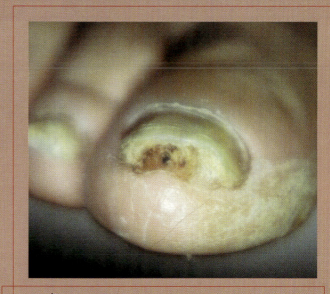

Onychomycosis (Tinea Unguium) [Fig. 5-17]

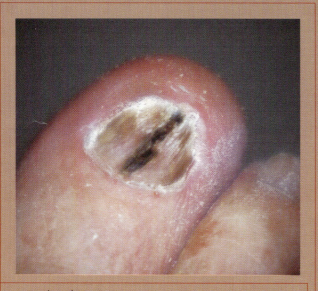

Fungal Infection [Fig. 5-18]

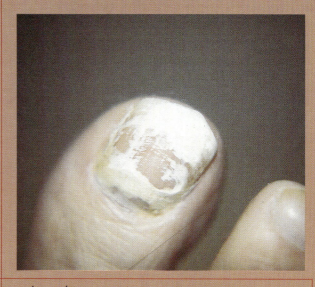

Leukonychia Mycotica [Fig. 5-19]

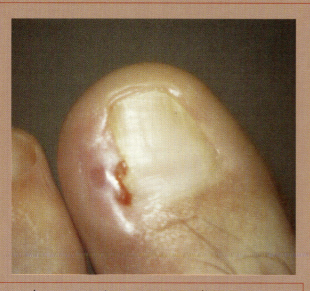

Onychocryptosis (Ingrown Toenail) [Fig. 5-21]

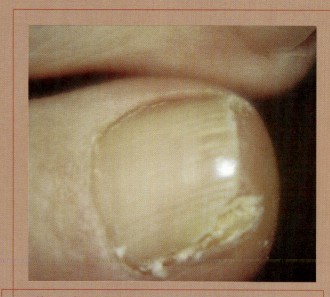

Calloused Nail Groove [Fig. 5-23]

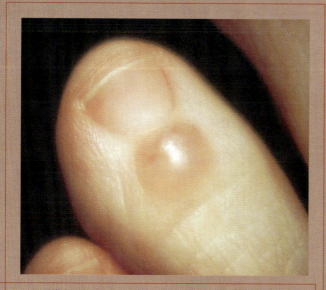

Mucoid Cyst [Fig. 5-25]

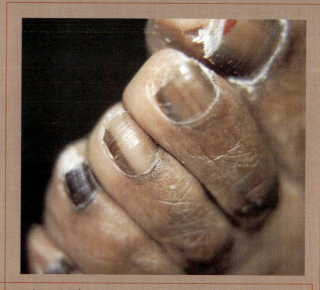

Melanonychia [Fig. 5-26]

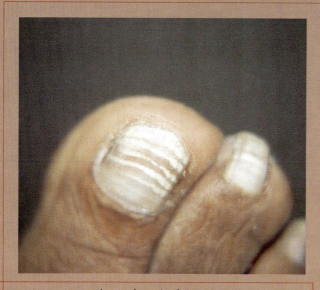

Transverse Leukonychia (White Lines) [Fig. 5-27]

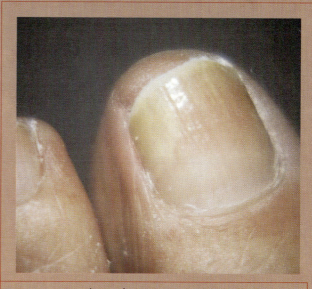

Apparent Leukonychia [Fig. 5-28]

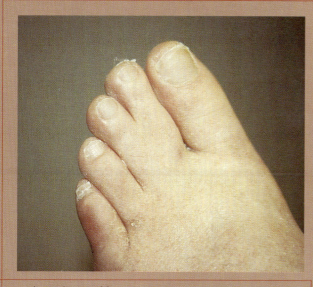

Syndactyly (Webbing) [Fig. 6-1]

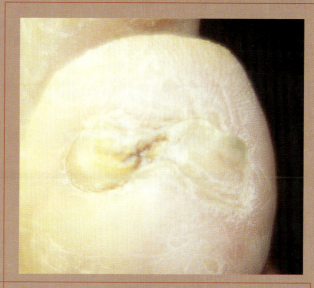

Synpolydactyly (Double Toenail) [Fig. 6-2]

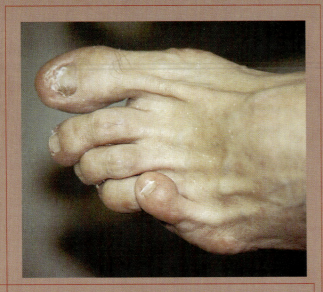

Digiti Quinti Varus [Fig. 6-3]

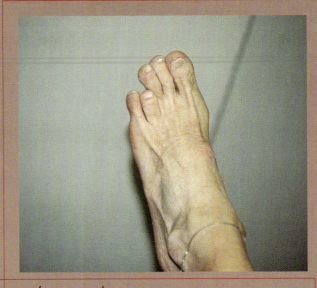

Brachymetapody [Fig. 6-4]

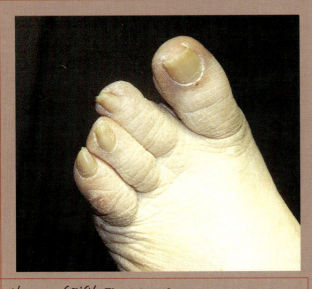

Absence of Fifth Toe [Fig. 6-6]

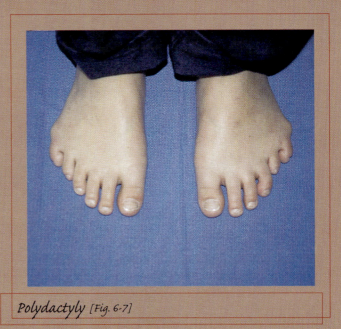

Polydactyly [Fig. 6-7]

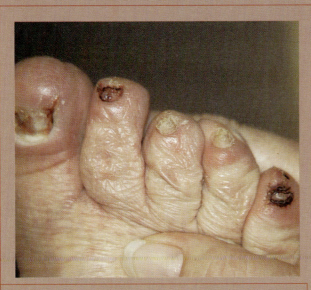

Onychotillomania [Fig. 6-9]

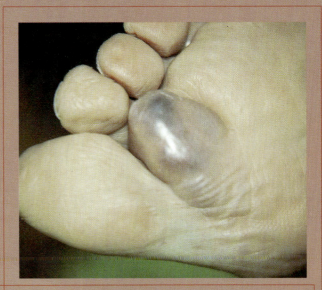

Telangiectatic Fibroma (Fibrous Tumor) [Fig. 6-12]

Answers to Chapter Review Questions

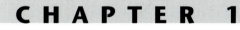

CHAPTER 1

1. The evolution of the longitudinal arch

2. The "Lotus Foot" because the foot after binding resembled the lotus flower.

3. The position assumed by the body when the individual stands erect with the head, eyes, and toes directed forward. The arms are by the sides of the body with the palms facing forward and the legs are together.

4. Because all terms describing the motions and relationships of body parts assume the body to be in that position.

5. The top

6. The bottom, the other term is the "sole" of the foot.

7. The tibia is the leg bone and it is located on the medial side of the leg.

8. The fibula is the leg bone and it is located on the lateral side of the leg.

CHAPTER 2

1. The calcaneous or heel bone

2. 19–20 on the bottom and one on the top

3. 1. The dorsalis pedis pulse, located on the top (dorsum) of the foot over the navicular and middle cuneiform bones. 2. The posterior tibial pulse which is located on the medial side (big toe side) of the foot below the tip of the medial malleolous.

4. An inflamed lymph vessel

5. Excess fluid within the tissue spaces

6. The integumentary system or skin. (It covers an area almost the size of a 9' x 12' rug!)

7. Collagen

8. Hair, nails, sweat glands, and sebaceous glands

CHAPTER 3

1. A disease that affects the entire body.

2. A systemic disease of unknown origin that affects the organ systems of the body by the abnormal deposition of collagen in the tissues. It is particularly noted in the skin, which loses its elasticity.

3. Inflammatory and noninflammatory arthritis; inflammatory arthritis causes destruction of bone and noninflammatory arthritis causes new bone formation.

4. Rheumatoid arthritis is inflammatory and osteoarthritis is noninflammatory.

5. Pain caused from a lack of oxygen to the tissues.

6. Two; it is estimated that there are 11 million known diabetics in the United States or 1 in 20.

7. Insulin is used to control type 1 diabetes.

8. The disease causes hardening of the arteries and those first affected are the arterioles.

9. Because diabetics as a result of the disease lose the feeling in their feet. They may sustain small injuries that they do not feel. If not cared for, these may become infected and be life-threatening.

1. It starts at heel strike and ends at the point at which the leg is aligned vertically, or at 90°, to the foot.

2. An orthotics is a prescription device prescribed by a doctor custom made from a neutral position cast of the patient's foot. An arch support is not made to a neutral position cast of the foot and may be purchased over the counter by anyone.

3. a. The left and right shoe lasts.
   b. The invention of the sewing machine.
   c. A system of shoe sizing by Edwin Simpson.

4. The difference in length between one size and another is only one-third of an inch.

5. It is the name for the mold over which a shoe is constructed.

6. If the skin of the area to be serviced is infected, inflamed, broken, or swollen the nail professional should not service the client. The author believes that in some cases of swelling a foot service may be safely performed.

7. It is the skin's attempt to protect itself from chronic irritation or injury.

8. There is no real difference other than where they are located. Corns are on the toes, a callus is generally found on the bottom of the foot or the heels.

9. A callus is not alive so there are no blood vessels found within the callus. Warts, because they are a true skin tumor, are alive and have many small blood vessels called capillaries. These capillaries may be seen as small red or black dots on the surface of the wart.

10. a. *Staphylococcus*
    b. *Streptococcus*
    c. *Pseudomonas*

11. Eccrine sweat glands are found on the sole of the foot. It is estimated there are over 600 of these glands in each square centimeter of the sole of the foot!

12. The evaporation of perspiration from the skin of the feet is, in most instances, the most common cause.

13. A Morton's neuroma is a scar formation around one of the plantar intermetatarsal nerves in the ball of the foot. The client will complain of a sharp pain, or cramp in the ball of the foot when walking or wearing shoes. The acute nature of the pain in the absence of obvious signs of other disease processes should be the tip that a neuroma is present.

CHAPTER 5

1. Matrix bed, cuticle (eponychium and hyponychium), nail plate, nail bed, specialized ligaments, and the nail folds

2. By understanding how the different structures of the nail module produce a normal nail plate it is easier to determine what structure or structures are involved with an abnormal nail plate. Once the location of the disorder is determined a probable cause is easier to identify.

3. Any disease or deformity of the nail

4. Onychomycosis

5. Tile-shaped nails and plicatured nails

6. Yes, as long as there is no infection present in the area.

7. Almost 100% show these black bands in their nails!

CHAPTER 6

1. A deviation from the average or norm, anything structurally unusual or irregular or contrary to a general rule

2. An uncontrollable urge to pick one's nails.

CHAPTER 7

1. Because it gives basic information necessary to set up records (computer or written) and helps begin the history and personal evaluation process.

2. Because you do not want to recommend or use products that the client may be allergic to.

3. Because some medical conditions will affect the services you recommend to the client, i.e., diabetes and poor circulation.

CHAPTER 8

1. Because of its porous nature it cannot be properly sanitized or disinfected.

2. Professional nail nippers (not the modified fingernail clippers), curette, small nail rasp, a regular nail file (diamond recommended for ease of disinfection), and a foot file or paddle

3. The shape of the toenail is more arched, side to side, than are fingernails. Trimming it in one cut causes the plate to flatten out and increases the incidence of the edges of the nail plate tearing free from the underlying hyponychium and nail bed.

4. The hand-held, the cable-driven, the belt-driven, and the micro-motor type. No, improper use of the drill by an untrained operator causes injury to the client.

5. Because if used properly it will produce less heat while cutting down the thickness of the nail.

CHAPTER 9

1. Because of the enclosed environment and the numbers of different people who visit the salon.

2. Sanitation—to clean, or to promote health as from the word sanitary. Disinfection—to free from pathogenic organisms or to make them inert or incapable of producing disease. Sterilization—the complete elimination of microbial viability.

3. Biocidal means against or destroying living organisms. Yes, disinfectants are biocidal agents. Because we are a living organism, we must be cautious when using disinfectant solutions.

4. Alcohols, iodoforms, quaternary ammonium compounds (QUATS), phenolics, and glutaraldehydes

5. You!

6. Washing your hands.

7. Only once! Make the most of it or they will probably not return for a second.

8. Because it is more efficient for you to give the pedicure when the client is elevated and clients equate an elevated chair with being more professional.

CHAPTER 10

1. Everyone!

2. Soaking agents, scrubbing agents, and massage preparations

3. Good grooming, and they are a preventive health aid that promotes foot health.

4. This depends on the health of the client. Around 104°F is the optimum temperature for healthy clients. No more than 100°F for clients with circulatory disorders or neuropathies in the lower extremities.

5. Reduce only enough callus to make the client comfortable. Remember a callus is nature's method of protecting the skin. A good rule of thumb is that callus should be "smoothed not removed."

6. It increases circulation of blood and lymph, and it relaxes the muscles.

7. Effleurage consists of light and hard stroking movements. Pétrissage is compression that includes kneading, squeezing, and friction movements. Effleurage relaxes muscles and improves circulation to the small surface blood vessels. Pétrissage promotes increased movement by stretching muscles, tendons, and scar tissues from previous injuries.

Further Reading Selections

CHAPTER 2

Charlesworth, F. (1961). *Chiropody Theory and Practice.* London: Actinic Press.

Gray, H. & Gross, C.M.(1985). *Gray's Anatomy.* Philadelphia: Lea & Febiger.

Mercado, O.A. (1972). *An Atlas of Podiatric Anatomy.* Chicago: National Academy Hospital Podiatry.

Moore, K.L. (1992). *Clinically Oriented Anatomy.* Baltimore: Williams & Wilkins.

Scali-Sheahan, M. (1994). *Milady's Human Anatomy and Physiology Workbook.* Albany, NY: Milady.

CHAPTER 3

Miller, B.F. & Keane, C.B. (1987). *Encyclopedia and Dictionary of Medicine, Nursing, and Allied Health* (4th ed.) Philadelphia: Saunders.

Robbins, J.M. (1994). *Primary Podiatric Medicine.* Philadelphia: Saunders.

Samitz, M.H. (1981). *Cutaneous Disorders of the Lower Extremities* (2nd ed.) Philadelphia: Lippincott.

Zier, B.G. (1990). *Essentials of Internal Medicine in Clinical Podiatry.* Philadelphia: Saunders.

CHAPTER 4

Coughlin, M. & Frey, C. (1994, May/June). Cruel Shoes. *Biomechanics,* 34.

Levine, S.M. (1991 May). High-Heeled Shoes and Foot Comfort, *Current Podiatric Medicine,* 17.

Mix, G.F. (1994, December). If the Shoe Fits. *Nails Magazine,* 40-46.

Robbins, J.M. (1994). *Primary Podiatric Medicine.* Philadelphia: Saunders.

Rossi, W.A. (1990, June). A Brief History of Footwear. *Current Podiatric Medicine,* 32.

Rossi, W.A. (1994, June). Shoe Sizes: The Big Bamboozle. *Podiatry Management,* 47.

Trevor, E. (1994 May/June). Simple Steps to Keep Your Feet in Walking Order—Feet First. *The Walking Magazine,* 47.

Women in Pain. (1994, May/June). Biomechanics, 39.

Yale, I. (1974). *Podiatric Medicine.* Baltimore: William & Wilkins.

CHAPTER 5

Baran, R., Barth, J., & Dawber, R. (1991). *Nail Disorders—Common Presenting Signs, Differential Diagnosis and Treatment.* New York: Churchill Livingstone.

Miller, B.F. & Keane, C.B. (1987). *Encyclopedia and Dictionary of Medicine, Nursing, and Allied Health* (4th ed.). Philadelphia: Saunders.

Scher, R.K., Daniel, C.R., III. (1990). *Nails: Therapy, Diagnosis, Surgery.* Philadelphia: Saunders.

Zaias, N. (1980). The Nail in Health and Disease. New York: SP Medical Books.

CHAPTER 7

Gross, R.H. (1948). *Modern Foot Therapy.* Modern Foot Therapy Publishing.

Seidel, H.M., Ball, J.W., Dains, J.E., & Benedict, G.W. (1987). *Mosby's Guide to Physical Examination.* St. Louis: Mosby.

Zier, B.G. (1990). *Essentials of Internal Medicine in Clinical Podiatry.* Philadelphia: Saunders.

CHAPTER 9

Aronoff, H., Neufeld, R.I., Karpo, A.S., Terleckyj, B., Axler, D.A. (1982). An Evaluation of the Fungicidal Activity of Disinfectants Commonly used in Clinical Practice. *Journal of the American Podiatry Association, 72,* 23.

Chesky, R., Cristina, I., Rosenberg, R.B. (1994). *Playing It Safe—Milady's Guide to Decontamination, Sterilization, and Personal Protection.* Albany, NY: Milady. (An excellent reference for the salon library)

Coleman, R. N. (1992, December). Disinfectants—An Overview of Disinfectants and Their Proper Use. *Podiatry Today,* 59.

Emmons, W., Binford, C.H., Utz, J.P. (1963). *Medical Mycology.* (Chap. 1, 2, 4, 10, 14) Philadelphia: Lea & Febiger.

Grahm, B. (1994, April). Beauty and Health—Make Sure your Manicure is Safe. *Glamour,* 82.

Industry News (1994, June). Texas Passes Tuberculocidal Requirement. *Nailpro,* 80.

Malack, P. (1991, March). How to Maintain That Cutting Edge (instrument care and cleaning). *Podiatric Products,* 64.

Malack, P. (1991, May). Another Look at Disinfectants and Sterilizing Solutions. *Podiatric Products,* 38.

McCormick, J. (1994, June). Clean Profits. *Nailpro,* 12,.

Owens, B. (1994, May). Understanding Disinfectants. *Nailpro,* 33.

Owens, B. (1994, June). Professional File Tabs—Cleaning and Storage. *Nailpro,* 79.

Salon Sanitation: for the Health of Your Business (1994, March). *Nails,* 26.

Schoon, D. (1994). *HIV/AIDS & Hepatitis—Everything You Need to Know to Protect Yourself and Others.* Albany, NY: Milady. (An excellent reference book)

Schoon, D. (1994, March). AIDS and Salon Disinfection. *Nails,* 42.

Smith, T., & Conant, N.F. (1960). *Zinsser Microbiology* (12th ed.) New York: Appleton-Century-Crofts. (Use as general reference)

Stewart, R.C. & Ayers, L.W. (1977). A Plea for more Rational Use of "Cold Sterilization" Procedures in Podiatric Medicine. *Journal of the American Podiatry Association, 67,* 441.

Terleckyj, B. & Axler, D.A. (1993). Efficacy of Disinfectants against Fungi Isolated from Skin and Nail Infections. *Journal of American Podiatry, 83,* 386.

CHAPTER 10

Beck, M. (1994). *Theory and Practice of Therapeutic Massage.* Albany, NY: Milady.

Dougans, I. (1996). *The Complete Illustrated Guide to Reflexology—Therapeutic Foot Massage for Health and Wellbeing.* Rockport, MA: Element Books.

Hess, S. (1996). *The Professional's Reflexology Handbook.* Albany, NY: Milady.

Milady (1997). *Milady's Art and Science of Nail Technology* (3rd ed.). Albany, NY: Milady.

Appendix of Sources

This is a partial list of suppliers of products that are related to the provision of foot services. I am familiar with these manufacturers and suppliers and recommend their products. For a more complete listing of manufacturers and suppliers please refer to *Nails Magazine-Fact Book* or *Nailpro Magazine-Gold Book*. Each of these is published once a year by the respective magazines and have complete listings of all manufacturers and suppliers of nail-related products.

AROMATHERAPY

Aroma Vera
5901 Rodeo
Los Angeles, CA 90016
Phone: 310/280-0407,   800/669-9514
FAX: 310/280-0395

Aveda Corporation
4000 Pheasant Ridge Dr.
Minneapolis, MN 55449
Phone: 612/783-4000, 800/283-3224
FAX: 612/783-4110

DISINFECTION & SANITATION PRODUCTS

Backscratchers
Salon Aseptic Control System
8120 Berry Ave., Ste. B
Sacramento, CA 95828
Phone: 916/381-8383, 800/832-5577
FAX: 916/381-7336

Ultronics
750 Corporate Dr.
Mahwah, NJ 07430
Phone: 201/512-8003, 800/262-6262
FAX: 201/529-2178

DISPLAY RACKS & CUSTOM PLASTIC PRODUCTS

Home Grown Creations
9909 Canoga Ave., Unit F
Chatsworth, CA 91311
Phone: 818/407-8859, 800/407-8859
FAX: 818/407-8837

DRILLS

Erica's Diamond Bits and Electric Files
ATA
261 East Broad St.
Westerville, OH 43081
Phone: 614/895-7181, 800/776-8324
FAX: 614/895-5423

Kupa
6980 Aragon Cir., Unit 6
Beauna Park, CA 90620
Phone: 714/739-2081, 800/994-5872
FAX: 714/739-2084

Medicool Inc.
23761 Madison St.
Torrance, CA 90505
Phone: 310/791-3746
FAX: 310/375-2219

INSTRUMENTS

Creative Nail Design Systems
(see Pedicure Supplies)

Erica's Diamond File
(See Drills)

Mehaz Worldwide/Charles G. Spilo
585 South Santa Fe Ave.
Los Angeles, CA 90013
Phone: 213/687-8600, 800/34-SPILO
FAX: 888/34-SPILO

Realys—Tropical Shine Files
7601 Woodwind Dr.
Huntington Beach, CA 92647
Phone: 714/842-1702, 800/4-REALYS, 800/473-2597
FAX: 714/848-0946

Tweezerman Corporation
55 Sea Cliff Ave.
Glen Cove, NY 11542
Phone: 516/676-7772, 800/645-3340
FAX: 516/676-7998

PEDICURE SUPPLIES

Amoresse Laboratories Inc.
4121 Buchanan St.
Riverside, CA 92503
Phone: 909/273-9400, 800/258-7931
Fax: 909/273-9506

Beautiful Feet
16632 Burke Ln.
Huntington Beach, CA 92647
Phone: 714/375-259, 800/656-2646
FAX: 714/375-2596

Creative Nail Design Systems
1125 Joshua Way
Vista, CA 92083
Phone: 619-599-2900, 800/833-NAIL
FAX: 619/599-4007

Estelina's Slipaway
31210 La Baya Dr. #211
West Lake Village, CA 91362
Phone: 818/879-5461, 800/745-FOOT
Fax: 818/879-1843

Gena Laboratories
P.O. Box 380459
Duncanville, TX 75138-0459
Phone: 214/296-2887, 800/233-4362
FAX: 214/296-4634

Salon Systems
2220 Gaspar Ave.
Los Angeles, CA 90040
Phone: 213/728-2999, 800/621-9585
FAX: 213/726-6271

SALON & PEDICURE EQUIPMENT

European Touch Ltd. II
P.O. Box 322
Brookfield, WI 53008-0322
Phone: 414/783-7016, 800/626-6912
FAX: 414/783-6306

Jeffco
5269 U.S. Highway 158
Advance, NC 27006
Phone: 910/998-8193, 800/951-8294
FAX: 910/998-5315

Kayline Enterprises
P.O. Box 90399
Long Beach, CA 90809
Phone: 310/595-4515, 800/821-3444, 800/237-7931 (CA)
FAX: 310/492-1292

Pibbs Industries
133-15 32nd Ave.
Flushing, NY 11354
Phone: 718/445-8046, 800/551-5020
FAX: 718/461-3910

Glossary/Index

Abduction—rotational motion of the leg in the horizontal or transverse plane causing the toes or distal aspect of the foot to move away from the median plane. 8, *fig. 1-1,* 61

Abraded—abrade, to wear down or rub away by friction; erode. 74

Abscesses—plural for abscess, a localized collection of pus in a cavity formed by the disintegration of the tissue. 82

Acupuncture—technique, as for relieving pain or inducing regional anesthesia, in which thin needles are inserted into the body at specific points. 199

Acute—having severe symptoms. 40

Adduction—rotational motion of the leg in the horizontal or transverse plane causing the toes or distal aspect of the foot to move toward the median plane. 8, *fig. 1-10,* 61-62

Adenovirus—large group of virus capable of causing disease in the upper respiratory tract. 171

Alcohols—a class of disinfectants whose active ingredient is usually isopropyl alcohol. There can be others such as ethyl, methyl, or benzyl alcohols. 172-173

Alpha-hydroxy acid, (AHA)—organic acid, naturally derived or synthetically produced, used in the beauty industry to help partially dissolve and soften the outer keratin layer of the skin. It is used in pedicure products to help soften and partially remove callus tissues on the foot. 188

Amelanotic—without melanin. 88

Anatomic position—that position assumed when a person stands erect with the head, eyes, and toes directed forward. The arms are by the sides of the body with the palms of the hands facing forward and the legs are together. 6, 10

Anemia—any condition in which the number of red blood cells or the amount of hemoglobin found in the red blood cells is less than normal. 34, 43-44

Aneurysm—a sac or dilation formed as the result of the weakening of the wall of an artery, vein, or the heart. 45

Anhydrosis—inability to produce sweat. 84-85

Anomaly—deviation from the average or norm, anything that is structurally unusual or irregular or contrary to a general rule. 131

Anterior—in general anatomic terms, refers to the front surface of the body. In the foot it refers to a part of the foot closer to the toes, i.e., the toe bones are anterior to the metatarsal bones. 18

Antioxidants—chemical compound or substance that inhibits oxidation. 188

Antiseptic—capable of preventing infection by inhibiting the growth of microorganisms. 22-24

Apparent leukonychia—nail plate appears white because of the abnormal refraction of light through the plate as the result of onycholysis, or because the tissues under the plate appear white. 127

Arch support—nonprescription device that supports the arch. It is generally purchased over the counter or by mail, according to shoe size or a foot impression. 64

Aromatherapy—use of selected fragrant substances in lotions and inhalants in an effort to affect mood and promote health. 188

Arteries—plural for artery, thick muscular-walled blood vessels that carry blood away from the heart to the tissues. 22-24

Arterioles—small arteries. 24

Arthritis—condition that causes swelling and inflammation of a joint with resultant pain. 37-41

Articulate—to join or connect together loosely to allow motion between parts. 15-16

Athlete's foot—see tinea pedis. 78

Atopic—hereditary predisposition toward the development of certain hyper-sensitivity reactions, such as hay fever, asthma, or skin reactions. 84

Atrophy—decrease in size, wasting, of a normally developed organ or tissue. 46

Autonomic—not subject to voluntary control, i.e., sweat production is an autonomic response. 84

Avulse—tearing away of a structure or part. 120

Bacteria—plural for bacterium, single-celled microorganisms. Many species present in nature. They multiply by cell division about every 20 minutes, which gives them a high geometric rate of population growth and evolution. Many species cause disease and infections in humans. 82-83, 171

Bacteriocidal—kills, destroys bacteria. 171

Beau's lines—transverse grooves or groove (not ridges) extending from one side of the nail plate to the other. 110-22, *fig. 5-7*

Bed epithelium—thin sheet of tissue between the nail bed and the nail plate. It originates from the distal matrix bed. This tissue is tightly attached to the plate and loosely attached to the nail bed. The bed epithelium has microridges that track in corresponding microgrooves on the nail bed. The bed epithelium, because of the strong attachment to the plate, slides along these grooves as the nail plate grows. 102

Benign—not malignant, harmless. 37

Biocidal—destroys living organisms. 172

Blood pressure—pressure the blood exerts against the walls of the blood vessels as the result of the heart contracting. The term usually refers to the pressure of the blood within the arteries (arterial blood pressure). It is measured with a blood pressure cuff called a sphygmomanometer. The pressure is recorded in millimeters of mercury (mm Hg). "Normal" blood pressure is said to be 120 mm Hg systolic (see definition) to 80 mm Hg diastolic (see definition). As we age the pressure increases somewhat; because of the aging process in the arteries and other tissues, they become less elastic. 23

Bone spurs—see exostosis. 41

Brachymetapody—visible shortness of the fingers or toes as the result of a congenitally short metacarpal or metatarsal. In the foot it seems to usually be the fourth toe as the result of a short fourth metatarsal. 132

Bromidrosis—foul-smelling perspiration. 72, 84

Bunion—an abnormal enlargement of bone on the inner aspect (medial) of the first metatarsal head. 38, 92-93

Callous or callus—thickening of the keratin layer of the skin as the result of repeated friction or intermittent pressure. Hard skin. Synonyms: keratoma, tyloma. 27, 73-75, *fig. 4-5*

Candida—a yeast-like fungus that is commonly part of the normal flora on humans and animals. It likes to live in warm moist areas and if the right circumstances arise will cause infections. 79

Capillary—small blood vessels within the tissues, single cell wall in thickness, that connect the arterioles and venules. The oxygen and nutrients are passed through the walls of these vessels into the surrounding tissues. 24

Capillary filling time—after applying pressure to an area of the skin to squeeze the blood out, it is the time it takes for the blood to return into that area of skin, which is noted by a return of the normal pinkish color. 56, 145

Carbolic acid—see phenol. 170, 172

Carrier—an individual who harbors (carries) a specific pathogenic organism of disease and is capable of transmitting that organism (disease) to others. 170

Catalyst—substance, usually used in small amounts relative to the reactants, that modifies and increases the rate of a reaction without being consumed in the process.

Charcot joint—a progressive relatively pain-free degeneration of the stress-bearing part of a joint as the result of neurologic disorders that cause a loss of sensation within the joint. 53-54

Chiropractor—one who practices a system of therapy in which disease is considered the result of abnormal function of the nervous system. The method of treatment usually involves manipulation of the spinal column and other body structures. 199

Chromonychia—color change in the nail. 126-28

Chronic—symptoms persisting for a long time, symptoms may become progressively worse over that period. 37

Chronologic—the number of years a person has lived. 141

-cidal—an adjective for -cide, a word element meaning an agent that kills or destroys. 171

Cirrhosis—disease of the liver characterized by a fibrous degeneration of the liver tissues. 85

Clavus—a corn. 75-76

Clubbing—a bulbous swelling of the ends of the fingers or toes giving them a club-like appearance. It is observed in various disease processes and its cause is unknown. 112

Collagen—fibrous structural protein that constitutes the protein of the white fibers of skin, tendon, bone cartilage, and all other connective tissues of the body. 29, 36

Communicator—one who can express himself in such a way that he is quickly and easily understood. 138

Configuration—arrangement of its parts, formation. 112

Contaminating—the introduction or possible introduction of an infectious agent onto a surface or into the body or some other liquid or material. 152

Contra-—word element meaning against or opposed.

Contracture—abnormal shortening of muscle or scar tissue, which results in distortion or deformity, especially of a joint of the body. 90

Corn—usually referring to a callus on the toe. See clavus, callus, heloma. 75-76, 123-24

Cornified—having become a horny formation. Synonym: keratinized. 102

Coronal or frontal planes—vertical planes that pass through the body or body part at right angles to the median plane. These planes divide the body or body part into front (anterior) and back (posterior) portions. 6, *fig. 1-6*

Curette—small scoop or spoon-shaped instrument, basically looks like a miniature melon baller. 155-56

Cuticle—narrow band of epidermis that extends onto the nail plate from the proximal nail fold. This is the distal part of the eponychium. 101

Cuticular system—folds of skin at the base of the nail plate that fold onto the nail plate and end on the plate as the eponychium or hyponychium. See eponychium, hyponychium. 101-2

Cyanosis—bluish discoloration of the skin and other tissues as a result of inadequate circulation to the tissues. The discoloration is due to an inadequate amount of oxygen in the blood and tissues. 35

Debilitation—generalized loss of strength, weakness. 79

Debridement—the removal of dead or dying tissue and debris from an area. 86

Denaturation—change in the usual nature of a substance, i.e., chemically splitting the molecular structure to destroy the substance or organism. 172

Dependent position—hanging down. 47

Dermatitis—inflammation of the skin. 85

Dermatophyte—any of various fungi that can cause parasitic skin infections. 171

Dermatophytosis—fungal infection of the skin. 78

Diabetes—any of several metabolic disorders marked by excessive discharge of urine and persistent thirst. 49-56

Diabetes insipidus—disorder characterized by the excessive production of urine, from 2 to 10 liters a day, while there is an increased intake of fluid that does not match the output of urine. It does not relate to any problems seen in the foot.

Diabetes mellitus—a complex disorder related to lack of or improper metabolism of insulin, which results in the improper metabolism of glucose, proteins, and fats. 50

> **Insulin-dependent diabetes mellitus (type 1, IDDM)**—requires the use of insulin to control blood sugars. At one time was termed juvenile diabetes. 50

> **Non–insulin dependent diabetes mellitus (type 2, NIDDM)**—does not require insulin to control blood sugars. At one time was termed adult-onset diabetes. 50-51

Diastolic—adjective for diastole, which is that period when the heart relaxes after contracting thus allowing the blood to flow back into the heart. 23

Diastolic pressure—the pressure measured in the artery when the heart is relaxed. 23

Dilate—to make wider or larger; cause to expand. 172-73

Diluent—inert substance used to dilute. 174

Disinfectant—agent that destroys infection-producing organisms, freeing from infection. 171, 176

Disinfection—to free from pathogenic organisms or to render them inert. 168

Distal—a position or part toward the toes. 7

Diuretic—an agent that promotes urine formation and excretion. 39

Dorsal—refers to the top of the foot, or to a part nearer to the top of the foot. 7, 20

Dorsiflexion—motion in the sagittal plane causing the foot or toes to move up toward the leg. 8, *fig. 1-8,* 61

Dwell time—amount of time the disinfectant is in contact with the organism or surface to be disinfected. 173-74

Dystrophic—any disorder due to defective or faulty nutrition. 108

Edema—an accumulation of excessive amounts of fluid in tissue spaces, cells, or cavities in the body. 26, 47

Effleurage—light or hard stroking movements used in massage. 195

Emboli—plural for embolus, a clot or other plug in a vessel. 48

Eminence—a projection or rounded elevation raised above the general level of the surrounding area of bone. 16

Emphysema—excessive accumulation of air in the tissues or organs of the body. This term is generally associated with a lung disease in which some of the air passages become plugged with mucus resulting in a loss of elasticity of the lung and the trapping of air in the lung tissues. 35

Endocarditis—inflammation of the inner lining (endocardium) of the heart. 42

Enzyme—any protein that acts as a catalyst to increase the rate at which a chemical reaction occurs. 172

Epidermis—the outermost layer of the skin. No blood vessels are found in this layer of the skin. 27-28

Eponychium—the most distal horny extension of the proximal nail fold. 30, 101

Ergonomic—adjective for ergonomics, the applied science of equipment design, as for the workplace, intended to maximize productivity by reducing operator fatigue and discomfort. 164

Erythrocyte—red blood cell; the red color is the result of the hemoglobin (see definition) carried within the cell. The hemoglobin carries the oxygen. 25

Etiology—the science and study of the causes of disease. 36

Eukaryotic—refers to eukaryote, which has to do with the make up of the cellular structure. Plants, animals, protozoa, fungi, and most forms of algas can be classified as being eukaryotic forms of life.

Eversion—The sole or plantar aspect of the foot moves in the frontal plane away from the midline or median plane of the body. 8, *fig. 1-13*, 61

Exfoliating—see exfoliative. 188

Exfoliative—detachment or shedding of the superficial cells from the surface of a tissue, in this case the skin. 84

Exostosis—a benign new growth of bone projecting from a bone surface. A bone spur. 41, 124

Facilitator—one who directs a conversation or discussion and makes it understandable and easy. 138

Fibroma—benign, usually enclosed, tumor composed primarily of fibrous tissue. 124

Fibular—refers to the nail margin or part of the foot toward the fibula, which is a bone on the outside or lateral aspect of the leg. It is on the same side of the leg as the little toe. The terms fibular and lateral can be used interchangeably. 8

Fissure—deep crack in the skin, a narrow slit or cleft. 75

Flora—the collective plant organisms of a given area or locality. 170

Friction blisters—a localized reaction of the skin to friction from an external source. 72-73

Fungi—any of numerous **eukaryotic** organisms of the kingdom Fungi, which lack chlorophyll and vascular tissue and range in form from a single cell to a body mass of branched filamentous **hyphae** that often produce specialized fruiting bodies. The kingdom includes the yeasts, molds, smuts, and mushrooms. 78-81, 171

Fungicidal—kills, destroys fungus. 173, 176

Gait cycle—This term refers to walking. A cycle starts from the point when the heel of one foot contacts the weight-bearing surface, through the point where the toe of the same foot leaves contact with the weight-bearing surface. 60-65

Gangrene—death of tissue usually associated with the loss of blood supply to those tissues. It may be localized to a small area, or it may involve an entire extremity or organ. 35

Genetic—relating to reproduction, birth or origin. Inherited. 45-131

Germinate—to cause to sprout or grow. 78

Glutaraldehydes—class of disinfectants. The aldehyde portion of these disinfectants is the active ingredient. This is the only class of disinfectants that is sporocidal; thus it may also be classed as a sterilizer. 172-73

Glycerin—clear, colorless, syrupy liquid, related to alcohols used as a solvent in drugs. In the pedicure scrubs it combines, like a solvent, with the flakes of skin and assists in the **exfoliating** process. 188

Gout—disorder of the metabolism in which excessive amounts of uric acid accumulate in the blood. The uric acid crystals are subsequently deposited in the joints and other tissues of the body resulting in sudden attacks of acute pain, swelling, and inflammation of the affected areas. This condition is frequently seen in the big toe joint. 34, 39

Gram negative—primary characteristic of a group of bacteria whose cell walls do not stain purple with Gram stain. 173

Gram positive—primary characteristic of a group of bacteria whose cell walls retain the purple Gram stain. 173

Gram stain—a staining method, using crystal violet stain, to quickly classify bacteria into two groups. 173

Hallux valgus—valgus means bent or twisted away from the midline of the body. Hallux valgus means that the great toe is rotated and abducted away from the midline of the body. 92-93

Hammertoe—condition of the toe in which the proximal phalanx is extended and the intermediate and distal phalanges are flexed, causing a claw-like appearance to the toe. 38, 90-91

Heloma—a corn. 75-76

Heloma durum—a hard corn, usually found over a joint on the toe. 75

Heloma molle—a soft corn, found between the toes where moisture causes the callus to become whitish in color, soft, and spongy in texture. 75

Hematoma—blood clot within the tissues. 115

Hemoglobin—chemical in the red blood cell that carries the oxygen; it is also what makes the red in the red blood cell. 25, 43

Hepatitis—inflammation of the liver from any cause. 171

HIV—human immunodeficiency virus. 171

Hominid—a small ape-like creature, our earliest direct ancestor, who walked in an upright manner on a foot almost identical to our own. 2, *fig. 1-1*

Horizontal or transverse planes—planes at right angles to both the median and coronal planes. These planes divide the part into a top and a bottom. In the foot the top is called the dorsal aspect and the bottom is the plantar aspect. 6, *fig. 1-7*

Hydrating—supplying water to a tissue or surface, assists in allowing water to penetrate the tissues. 188

Hydrostatic—relating to the pressure of fluids. 26

Hygiene—science that deals with the promotion and preservation of health. Conditions and practices that serve to promote or preserve health. 82

Hyphae—any of the threadlike filaments forming the living parts of a fungus.

Hyperhidrosis—excessive formation of perspiration, sweat. 83-84

Hyperkeratotic—an adjective for hyperkeratosis, which means an increase in the horny layer of the skin, or any disease process characterized by this process.

Hypertension—persistently high blood pressure. An adult is termed to have hypertension if the systolic pressure is 140 or higher and the diastolic pressure is 90 or higher. 43, 45

Hyponychium—area under the free edge of the nail where it attaches to the horny layer of skin. It is like the eponychium only is at the distal end of the nail module. 30, 101-2, 114

Hypoxia—deficiency in the amount of oxygen reaching body tissues. 112

Immune—being highly resistant to a disease as a result of the formation of antibodies by the system. 36

Immunodeficiency—deficiency of the immune response to infections. 128

Ingrown toenail—see onychocryptosis. 2, 4

Inorganic—nonliving, lacks carbon atoms within its structure. 106

Insensitive—without sensation or feeling. 53-54

Insulin—hormone normally produced in the pancreas by areas of tissue called the islets of Langerhans. This hormone is responsible for regulating the amount of glucose and other nutrients within our blood. Without it the glucose is not transported from the blood through the vascular membranes into the tissues where the glucose can be used by the body for energy. The lack of or improper metabolism of insulin therefore causes a state called diabetes. 50

Interdigital—between the fingers or toes. 88

Intermediate—means between two structures. 7

Intermittent claudication—group of symptoms, mainly characterized by pain in the calf muscles of one or both legs. Pain is brought on by walking and relieved by resting for a few minutes. The cause is blockage, partial or complete, of the main arteries supplying blood to the muscles of the leg. 35, 46-47

Inversion—the sole or plantar aspect of the foot moves in the frontal plane toward the midline or median plane of the body. 8, *fig. 1-12*, 61-62

Iodophors—disinfectants in which the active ingredient is iodine. 172-73

Ischemic—deficiency of blood in a part. 46

-itis—word element, refers to inflammation, i.e., bursitis means inflammation of a bursa.

Keratin—a protein that is the principle constituent of epidermis, nails and hair. 106

Keratinization—the development of keratin. 28

Keratoderma—a generalized thickening of the horny layer of the skin. 88

Ketoacidosis—excessive breakdown of protein or muscles within the body, which is potentially life threatening, and may in some cases be the initial symptom of type 1 diabetes. 50

Koilonychia—spoon-shaped nails. 112

Lamellar—splitting or peeling a thin scale, plate, or layer. 111

Last—block or form shaped like a human foot and used in making or repairing shoes. The form or mold over which a shoe is constructed. 66

Lateral—away from the median plane or center of the part. 7

Layperson—a nonprofessional, one who is not trained in a particular profession.

Lesion—any pathologic opening of the tissue. An ulcer or a sore can be termed a lesion. 39

Leukocyte—white blood cell, these fight infections within the body. 25

Leukonychia—white nail plate. 126-27

Leukonychia mycotica—whitish fungal infection on the top of the nail plate. 117, *fig. 5-19*

Lipophilic—affinity for fat, combine with or dissolve in fat. 176

Longitudinal—running lengthwise in the direction of the long axis of the body or any of its parts. 17-18, 110-12

Lunula—a whitish colored, moon-shaped area, seen under the nail plate just distal to the eponychium. It is the visible portion of the matrix bed. 30, 101

Lymph—transparent, slightly yellow to opalescent fluid found in the lymph vessels. It is about 95% water with some proteins and other components contained within the liquid portion of the blood. The main cellular components found in lymph are the white blood cells called lymphocytes. 25

Lymphangitis—inflammation of a lymph vessel. 26

Lymphatic—pertaining to lymph or a lymph vessel. 25, 147

Lysis—destruction, decomposition, or digestion, of a substance or organism. Often used with a prefix denoting the substance digested. 172

Macro—large scale, the opposite of micro.

Malady—disease, disorder, or ailment.

Malaise—general feeling of uneasiness or discomfort. Often the first sign of an infection or other disease process. 43

Malformation—abnormal formation or structure; a deformity. 112-13

Mallet toe—a condition of the toe in which the distal phalanx is flexed on the intermediate phalanx at the distal interphalangeal joint causing the toe to appear mallet-like. 91-92

Manipulation—skillful treatment by the hands. 195

Mask—cosmetic preparation that is applied to a body part and allowed to dry, either partially or totally, before being removed, used especially for cleansing and tightening, and invigorating the skin. 189-90

Massage—method of manipulation of the body that includes rubbing, pinching, kneading, or tapping. 195

Matrix bed—portion of the nail module that produces the nail plate. 30, 101

Medial—toward the median plane or center of the part. 7, 17

Medial malleolus—the bony bump on the medial side (big toe side) of the ankle. It is a part of the leg bone called the tibia. 24

Median plane—divides the body into equal left and right halves. It passes through the center of the body from front to back and from top to bottom. The median plane of the foot would pass through the middle of the third toe to the middle of the heel thus dividing the foot into two equal halves. 6, *fig. 1-4*

Melanocyte—pigment cell capable of producing melanin, a brown or black pigment. 28, 125

Melanoma—malignant lesion, usually of the skin, arising from the cells that are capable of forming melanin. The "black mole" or nevus of the skin. 87-88, *fig. 4-15,* 125-26

Melanonychia—black color seen in the nail caused by the production of melanin by melanocytes. 125, 127-28

Metabolism—complex of physical and chemical processes occurring within a living cell or organism necessary for the maintenance of life. 52

Micro—small scale, the opposite of macro. 152

Mold—any group of fungi that cause a dry cottony growth on organic substances. The color of the growth will depend on the species of fungi causing it. Many different colors are found. 78, 171

Molecular—see molecule. 189

Molecule—the smallest particle into which an element or a compound can be divided without changing its chemical and physical properties. 189

Monilia—see candida. 79

Morton's neuroma—see neuroma. 95-96, *fig. 4-21*

Nail bed—area to which the nail attaches as it grows beyond the matrix bed; the attachment of the plate to the bed is accomplished by the bed epithelium. 30, 101-2, 114

Nail folds—folds of skin along the sides of the nail plate, which form the nail grooves. 101-2

Nail module—is composed of six basic parts: matrix bed, nail bed, cuticular system ("cuticle," eponychium, and hyponychiun), nail plate, specialized ligaments, and the nail folds. These structures together are also called the nail unit. 101, *fig. 5-1*

Nail plate—visible hard portion of the nail module. 101, *fig. 5-1*

Naturopath—one who practices naturopathy, system of therapy that relies on natural remedies, such as sunlight supplemented with diet and massage, to treat illness. 199

Neuralgia—pain in or along a nerve. Usually sharp spasm-like pain that may occur at intervals. Generally caused from an inflammation or injury to the nerve. 44

Neurofibroma—see neuroma. 95-96, *fig. 4-21*

Neurogenic—originating in the nervous system. Forming nervous tissue or stimulating nerve energies. 37

Neurology—medical science that deals with the nervous system and disorders affecting it. 199

Neuroma—a nerve tumor, in the foot they are generally not a true neuroma but a fibrous scarring around the nerve referred to as a Morton's neuroma. 95-96

Neuropathy—a general term applied to functional disturbances and pathologic changes in the peripheral nervous system. 52-53

Nevus—nonmalignant localized overgrowth of melanin-forming cells of the skin present at birth or forming early in life. A mole. 86-87, *fig. 4-14*

Occlusion—obstruction or closing off, a blockage. 45

Onych(o)—word element referring to the nails. 109

Onychalgia—pain in the nails. 109

Onychitis—inflammation of the matrix of the nail. 109

Onychocryptosis—an ingrown toenail. 121-23

Onychodermal band—also called the solehorn, a thickened cornified band of tissue at the distal end of the nail plate where the bed epithelium meets the hyponychium. It can be visualized as a gray band, just before the free edge of the nail plate, by applying light pressure on the nail plate. 102

Onychodystrophy—malformation of the nail. 109

Onychoheterotopia—abnormal location of the nails. 109

Onychoid—resembling a fingernail or toenail. 110

Onycholysis—nail plate becomes detached from the nail bed, usually from the free edge, and can even become detached from the matrix bed under certain circumstances. 107, 116

Onychomadesis—shedding of the nail plate starting from the matrix bed. 115, *fig. 5-16*

Onychomycosis—fungal infection of the nail module. The most common disorder of the toenail. 116-19

Onychopathy—any disease or deformity of the nail. 110

Onychorrhexis—disorder of the nail plate seen as a series of narrow parallel grooves extending from the hyponychium to the free edge. 110, *fig. 5-6*

Onychoschizia—splitting of the nail plate in layers. 111-12

Onychosis—onychopathy. 110

Onychotillomania—a pathologic urge to pick the nails. 134

Onychotomy—incision or cutting into a nail. 110

Oral glucose tolerance test—laboratory test used to help make the diagnosis of diabetes mellitus. 51

Organ—any part of the body exercising a specific function. 14

Organic—having properties associated with living organisms. Organic materials all contain carbon atoms as part of their basic structure. 106

Orthotic—a true orthotic is a prescription device made to a neutral position cast of the foot. It allows for normal foot motions and stops abnormal motions. 64

Osteopath—one who practices osteopathy, a system of medicine based on the theory that disturbances in the musculoskeletal system affect other bodily parts, causing many disorders that can be corrected by various manipulative techniques in conjunction with conventional medical, surgical, pharmacologic, and other therapeutic procedures. 199

Oxygenation—saturation of tissues with oxygen. 42

Palpate—to examine by feeling or touching. 23

Pancreas—organ located behind the stomach. It assists in food digestion and is responsible for the production of insulin. 50

Papilloma—a wart. 76-78

Paralysis—a loss or impairment of motor function resulting from a wide variety of causes from injuries to disease to emotional disorders. It is not a disease process in itself. 44

Paronychia—inflammation of the soft tissue folds surrounding the nail plate. 119-21

Pasteurization—act or process of heating a beverage or other food to a specific temperature for a specific period of time to kill microorganisms that could cause disease, spoilage, or undesired fermentation. 170

Pathogenic—capable of causing disease. 169

Peripheral— on the surface or outer part of the body or organ.

Periungual—tissues or area around the nail plate. 110

Pes—refers to the foot. 89-90

Petechiae—minute, pinpoint, round, purplish red spots caused by bleeding within the skin or mucous membranes. Often part of a disease process. 43

Pétrissage—compression movements used in massage, which include kneading, squeezing, and friction. 195

pH—a measure of the degree to which a solution is acid or alkaline. On the pH scale 7 is the number determined to be a neutral pH. 174, *fig. 9-1*

Phagocytize —engulfing and ingestion of bacteria or other foreign bodies by phagocytes (white blood cells, erythrocytes). 25, 52

Phenol—an extremely poisonous compound derived from distilling coal tar or synthetically produced. It is used as an antiseptic and is one of the classes of disinfectants. Absorption through the skin causes colic, weakness, collapse, and local irritation; it is corrosive to metals. 170

Phenol coefficient—a measure of the bactericidal activity of a chemical compound in relation to phenol. Phenol is always 1 on the activity scale, everything else is less than 1. 172-73

Phenolics—class of disinfectants whose active ingredient is phenol; also known as carbolic acid. 172

Physiologic—basic processes of life, the functions of a living organism. 141

Pictograph—picture representing a word or idea. 199

Pincer nail—see trumpet nail. 113

Plantar—refers to the bottom of the foot or a part nearer to the bottom of the foot. 7, 20-21

Plantar wart—wart on the bottom of the foot. 76-78

Plantarflexion—motion in the sagittal plane causing the foot or toes to move down or away from the leg. 8, *fig. 1-9*, 61-62

Plasma—liquid portion of blood. 24

Platelet—see thrombocyte. 25

Plicatured nail—folded nail, the nail margin is folded at an angle down into the nail groove. 113

Pneumatic—pertaining to air, in this case run by air. 152

Polydactyly—multiple fingers or toes. 133

Polydipsia—excessive thirst. 50

Polyphagia—excessive intake of food. 50

Polyuria—excessive production of urine. 50

Porous—admitting the passage of gas or liquid through the substance.

Portal of entry—an avenue of entrance. For this context it is an opening in the skin or other tissues that allows for the entry of infectious bacteria, fungi, or other materials into the body. 82, 170

Posterior—in general anatomic terms this refers to the back surface of the body. In the foot it refers to a part of the foot that is closer to the heel, i.e., the metatarsal is posterior to the toe bones. 18

Precipitation—the settling of solid particles of a substance in solution. 39, 172

Pronation—is a complex triplane (taking place in three different body planes) motion consisting of simultaneous movement of the foot in the directions of abduction, eversion, and dorsiflexion. 8, *fig. 1-15*, 61

Prophylaxis—prevention of or protective treatment for disease. 118

Proximal—position or part toward the heel. 7

Psoriasis—noncontagious inflammatory skin disease characterized by recurring reddish patches covered with silvery scales. 88-89, *fig. 4-16*

Pterygium—a wing-like structure. In the foot it is seen as an abnormal adherence of the skin to the nail plate. Usually as a result of an injury to that area exhibiting this abnormal condition. (This term should not be confused with the term "cuticle.") 36, 107, 114

Pus—generally watery, yellowish-white fluid formed in infected tissue, consisting of white blood cells, cellular debris, and dead tissue. 25

Quaternary ammonium compounds (QUATS)—class of disinfectants whose available ammonium or chloride portions are the active ingredients. 172-73, 177

Reflexes—plural for reflex, meaning an involuntary action or response to external stimuli. 198

Reflexology—precise manipulation of the nerve endings in the hands and feet to stimulate the body's organs, nerves, and glands. 198-202

Ringworm—see dermatophytosis. 78

Sagittal planes—multiple planes that run parallel to the median plane. They differ from the median plane in that they do not divide the body or body part into equal halves. 6, *fig. 1-5*

Sanitization—to clean, as one would eating or drinking utensils. This word is derived from the word sanitary, which is defined as promoting or pertaining to health. 168

Saprophytes—organisms that live on dead or diseased organic matter. 116

SBE—subacute bacterial endocarditis. 43

Sciatic nerve—largest nerve in the body, it originates in the low back from a number of nerve roots from the spinal cord and its branches extend all the way down to the foot. 22, 63

Sclerotic—adjective for sclerosis, meaning a hardening of the tissues, especially the vascular system as well as the nervous system. 46

Sebaceous gland—glands found in the skin, produce an oily, colorless, odorless fluid (sebum). The opening of these glands are found in the hair follicles. 30

Sebum—the oily secretion of the sebaceous glands. 30

Silicone—any of a group of semi-inorganic polymers based on the structural unit R_2SiO, where R is an organic group, characterized by wide-range thermal stability, high lubricity, extreme water repellence, and physiologic inertness. 189

Soku Shinjutsu—Japanese for observation of the feet and treatment of the foot nerves. 199

Solehorn—see onychodermal band. 102

Soluble—capable of being dissolved. 39

Spasticity—state of increased muscle tone along with exaggerated deep tendon reflexes. 44

Specialized ligaments—attach the nail bed and matrix bed to the underlying bone. 101-2

Sphygmomanometer—an instrument used to measure blood pressure. 23

Spina bifida—congenital defect in which the spinal column is imperfectly closed so that part of the spinal cord protrudes, often resulting in neurologic disorders. 90

Splinter hemorrhages—small dark lines of dried blood, resembling splinters, which may be seen under the nail plate. They are this shape because they form along the microgrooves on the top of the nail bed. They are generally caused from minor injuries. 108, 114-15

Spore—small, usually single-celled reproductive body that is highly resistant to drying and heat and is capable of growing into a new organism. Spores are produced especially by certain bacteria, fungi, algae, and nonflowering plants. Spores have a hard outer shell like an egg. 78-79

Sporicidal—kills, destroys spores. 173, 176

Stasis—a stoppage or diminution of flow, as of blood or other body fluids. 42

Sterilization—process that completely eliminates all microbial viability (life). 169

Subacute—somewhat acute, between acute and chronic. 43

Subungual—tissues or area under the nail plate. 110, 115

Supination—complex triplane (taking place in three different body planes) motion consisting of simultaneous movement of the foot in the directions of adduction, inversion, and plantarflexion. 8, *fig. 1-14,* 62

Surfactant—surface-active substance such as soap or a synthetic detergent, a wetting agent. 188

Syndactyly—congenital or surgical webbing of the fingers or toes. In the foot, this condition is most commonly seen between the second and third toes. Some surgical procedures to correct hammertoes require surgical webbing to be part of the procedure. 132

Syndrome—combination of symptoms resulting from a single cause. 37

Synovial membrane—innermost lining of the joint capsule. This membrane secretes synovial fluid, which helps to lubricate the joint. 17

Synpolydactyly—a congenital condition in which an extra digit is completely webbed (syndactylized) to a normal digit. 132

Systemic—pertaining to or affecting the body as a whole. 34

Systolic—adjective for systole, that period during the contracture of the heart muscle that forces the blood into the blood vessels. 23

Systolic pressure—pressure measured in an artery when the heart is contracted. 23

Tapotement—percussion manipulation massage technique where the sides of the hands are used to strike the skin and underlying tissues in rapid succession. 196

Tea tree oil—an oil produced from the *Melaleuca alternifolia* tree. It has natural antiseptic qualities and is effective against fungus. 188

Telangiectatic—refers to telangiectasia, meaning a dilated capillary, artery, or vein on the surface of the skin. 135

Thrombocyte—also known as platelets, these assist in blood clotting. 25

Tibial—refers to the nail margin or part of the foot toward the tibia, a bone of the leg. It is on the same side of the leg as the big toe. The terms tibial and medial can be used interchangeably. 7

Tinea pedis—fungal infection of the skin of the foot, see dermatophytosis. 78

Tinea unguium—see onychomycosis. 116-19

Tophi—plural for tophus, a chalky white deposit of sodium urate crystals occurring in gout. 40

Transverse—crosswise, lying across the long axis of the body or any of its parts. 18, 110-11

Traumatic—a wound or injury, especially damage resulting from external force. 41

Trophic—pertinent to nutrition.

True cuticle—that part of the proximal nail fold, proximal to the hyponychium and lying immediately over the matrix bed, which is directly attached to the nail plate. It helps to seal the nail to the skin to keep out infection and foreign material. 101

Trumpet nail—disorder in which the edges of the nail plate originate parallel to each other but as they grow toward the free edge of the nail they curl around to form the shape of a trumpet at the free edge. 113

Tuberculocidal—kills or destroys the tubercule bacillus which causes tuberculosis. 176

Tyloma—see callous. Generally refers to a callus on the bottom of the foot. 73-75, *fig. 4-5*

Ungual—pertaining to the nails. 110

Vaccinia—viral disease of cattle commonly called cow pox. When communicated to man it usually produces an immunity to smallpox. 171

Vasoconstriction—narrowing of the blood vessel as a result of muscle contractions within or around the vessel. 94

Veins—thin-walled blood vessels that carry blood from the tissues back to the heart.

Venules—small veins. 24

Verruca—a wart. 76-78

Viability—capable of living. 169

Virucidal—kills, destroys virus. 173, 176

Virus—a unique class of infectious agents that are unable to reproduce outside of a living host cell. 171

Wart—hard, rough lump growing on the skin, caused by infection with certain viruses and occurring typically on the hands or feet. 76-78, 124

Yeast—general term for single-celled, usually round, fungi. Some yeasts are used for fermentation in alcohol production, others in the making of bread, and still others are pathogenic in man (candida, monilia). 78, 171

Zone therapy—pressures applied to particular zones of the body will cause a beneficial reflex action in another part of the same zone. 199